Pediatric
Basic Trauma Life Support

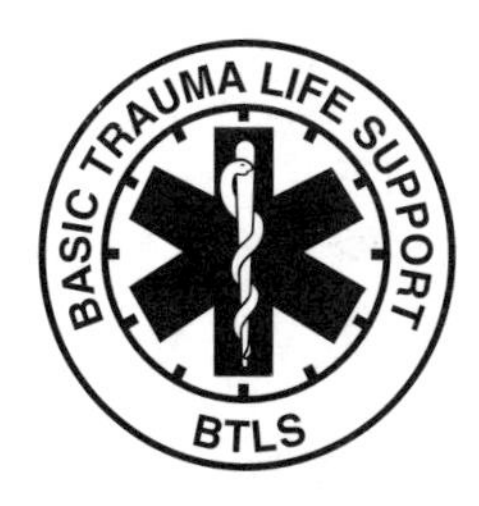

Anne Marie Dietrich, MD
Steven Shaner, EMT-P and
John Campbell, MD, FACEP, Editor
Ohio Chapter
American College of Emergency Physicians

Disclaimer

Basic Trauma Life Support International, Inc. makes every effort to ensure that contributors to its publications are knowledgeable authorities in their field. Readers are nonetheless advised that the statements and opinions expressed in this book are provided as guidelines and should not be construed as BTLS policy unless specifically referred to as such. BTLS disclaims any liability or responsibility for the consequences of any actions taken in reliance on those statements or opinions. The materials contained herein are not intended to establish policy, procedure or standard of care.

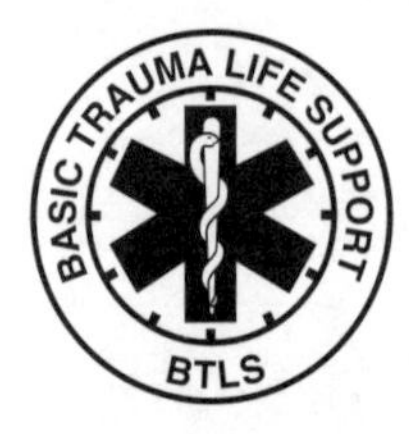

Basic Trauma Life Support International, Inc.
1 S. 280 Summit Avenue
Court B-2
Oakbrook Terrace, IL 60181

Additional copies of this publication can be ordered from BTLS International at 800-495-BTLS.

ISBN 0-9647418-1-4

10 9 8 7 6 5 4 3 2 1

Printed in the USA.

Cover Design:
Ryan J. Diersing
Whittier Elementary School
Westerville, Ohio

Selected Photos:
Denny Swick
Children's Hospital
Columbus, Ohio

Selected Graphics:
LifeART Images
Copyright 1994 Techpool Studios Corp. USA

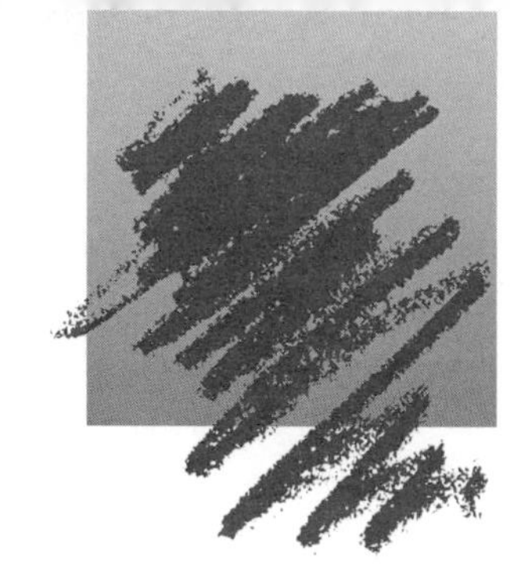

Contents

Forward

There is nothing so tragic as the death of a child. For a child who dies of injuries, this tragedy often has a devastating effect, not only on family and friends, but also on those EMS personnel who tried to save the child. For most of us in the EMS business, there is nothing that we dread more than to have to care for a critically injured child. Since trauma is the number one cause of death in children, we all must face this situation at some time. Unfortunately, most of us don't treat injured children often enough to develop the kind of expertise that we desire.

In 1982 the Basic Trauma Life Support course was developed to fill a void in the training for adult trauma care. Though care of the pediatric patient is taught in the BTLS course, everyone has been aware that there is much more to know about the injured child than can be covered in one chapter in an already intensive course. Pediatric trauma care is unique in several ways. Not only must you learn how to communicate with various ages of pediatric patients, but you also must learn how to communicate with the parents that accompany them. Because children's anatomy and activities are different than adults, they suffer different injuries. Assessment of the small child is often extremely difficult because the patient is frightened and struggling, can't communicate verbally, and has vital signs that are not only difficult to obtain but whose normal ranges are unfamiliar to us. Add to this an emotional parent and the job becomes almost overwhelming.

For several years, the international faculty of BTLS have discussed the need for an additional course to cover the special needs of the injured child. While PALS and APLS are excellent courses for pediatric emergencies, they do not devote enough time to pediatric trauma. In 1993 Ann Dietrich, MD, and Steve Shaner, EMT-P, with the support of the Ohio Chapter of the American College of Emergency Physicians and Ohio BTLS, accepted the challenge of producing a one-day course devoted to pediatric trauma care. The first draft was finished in 1994 and the course was field tested and rewritten many times over the next 18 months. After innumerable hours of work by Ann, Steve and many BTLS faculty, Pediatric BLTS was completed. The course is intended for EMS providers who have already had BTLS or PHTLS training and are familiar with adult trauma care. Pediatric BTLS provides necessary information about pediatric trauma, but its main focus is on the practical training needed to make you feel confident and competent when faced with caring for the critically injured child.

Due to the overwhelmingly positive response this course has received, this updated edition has been created. Several significant text changes have occurred, specifically in the areas of the assessment survey and hyperventilation in the child with head injuries. We hope you'll find this updated text reflective of recent policy changes in the treatment of children.

John E. Campbell, MD, FACEP
March, 1998

Authors

Nancy Asp, RN, MSN
MedFlight
Columbus, Ohio

James J. Augustine, M.D., FACEP
1994-95 President, Ohio Chapter ACEP
Premier Health Care Services
Dayton, Ohio

Bonnie L. Beaver, M.D., FACS, FAAP
Marshall University, School of Medicine
Department of Surgery
Chief of the Division of Pediatric Surgery
Huntington, West Virginia

William Cotton, M.D.
Department of Ambulatory Pediatrics
Children's Hospital
Columbus, Ohio

Lori Dandrea, M,.D.
Toledo, Ohio

Sharon Deppe, RN
Grant Medical Center
Columbus, Ohio

Ann M. Dietrich, M.D., FAAP, FACEP
Assistant Professor, Ohio State University
Education Medical Director, Ohio Chapter ACEP
Attending Physician, Children's Hospital
Ohio BTLS State Medical Director
Columbus, Ohio

Robert E. Falcone, M.D., FACEP
MedFlight Co-Medical Director
Grant Medical Center
Columbus, Ohio

Jeanette Foster, MSW
Children's Hospital
Child Abuse Team
Columbus, Ohio

Kathy Haley, BSN, CEN
Trauma Nurse Coordinator
Children's Hospital
Columbus, Ohio

Holly Herron, MSN
MedFlight
Columbus, Ohio

Sharon Hammond, RN, EMT-B
MedFlight
Columbus, Ohio

Jeffrey Kempf, D.O., FAAP
Attending Physician
Children's Hospital Medical Center of Akron
Division Emergency/Trauma Services
E.M.S. Medical Director
Akron, Ohio

David P. Keseg, M.D., FACEP
Columbus Division of Fire Medical Director
Premier Health Care Services
Columbus, Ohio

Laurie Lint, RN, EMT-P
Children's Hospital Medical Center of Akron
E.M.S. Coordinator/Educational Consultant
Division of Emergency/Trauma Services
Akron, Ohio

Linda Manley, RN, BSN, EMT-P
EMS Coordinator
Children's Hospital
Columbus, Ohio

Ronald McWilliams, NREMT-P
Assistant Director of Training
Southeast Ohio EMS, Inc.
Gallipolis, Ohio

Janet Metzger, RN
Columbus, Ohio

Nancy B. Nelson, MSW, LISW
Children's Hospital
Columbus, Ohio

Richard N. Nelson, M.D., FACEP
1992-93 President, Ohio Chapter ACEP
Ohio State University Hospitals
Columbus, Ohio

Randy L. Orsborn, NREMT-P
State BTLS Coordinator
Mount Vernon Fire Department
Flight Paramedic, MedFlight
Columbus, Ohio

Steve Shaner, EMT-P
Ohio BTLS Advisory Board
Grandview Heights Division of Fire
Flight Paramedic MedFlight
Columbus, Ohio

Katherine Shaner, RN, CEN, EMT-B
Transport Clinician
Children's Hospital
Columbus, Ohio

Howard A. Werman, M.D., FACEP
MedFlight Co-Medical Director
Ohio State University
School of Medicine
Columbus, Ohio

The Injured Child

Katherine Shaner, RN, CEN, EMT-B

Introduction

Today's health care providers are faced with caring for children from different backgrounds, races, and religions. In order to provide care in such a diverse world, care givers must learn to interact with children from all backgrounds. Communication is the key to providing excellent care to children and their families. Unlike adults, children have very different ways of communicating and making the "big" world understand them. They also have somewhat different fears and stressors than adults.

When dealing with sick or injured children, health care providers need to remember an important concept: We must treat not only the child, but also the family. Often it is difficult to remember that the child comes with an extra package – his parents and other family members.

Family–centered care is an ideal formed around the concept that a child's family is the constant in his life. Facilitating parent/professional collaboration and honoring cultural/ethnic diversity will enable health care providers to greatly enhance the medical experience for a child and the family.[1] The principle of family–centered care is that families need to be involved with the care of their children. According to Dr. Donald Brunquell of Minnesota Children's Hospital, "A family that feels explicitly involved is less likely to react in anger to fear and can be of great support to the child." Parents who are incorporated in the child's care will be much less frightened and more willing to provide pertinent information about the child, and comfort to the child, than those who are pushed to the side.

Basic communication skills are invaluable in health care situations and make parents feel that they are part of the "team" making a difference for their child. We must remember that parents feel responsible for their children, and it is their job to help and protect them. When a child is injured and the health care system takes over, parents are powerless and feel that they are not in control. Including parents in the care (i.e.,"Would you like to ride in the ambulance with Billy to the hospital? He needs you to be with him right now.") gives them back a sense of control.

The child's communication techniques and stressors are divided according to age groups. The following text explains these groups.

INFANCY

Infancy is the time between birth and 12 months. It is a time of rapid change and growth. By age 3 months, the infant will smile, make eye contact, and coo. An infant also will react to a care giver's voice and will follow visual stimuli. The infant will suck strongly and may hold a rattle briefly. As the child gets older, he learns to ambulate, first sitting (6 months), then crawling (9 months), and then walking (1 year).

Table 1.1 outlines developmental issues, fears, and techniques for different age groups.

Age (Yr)	Important Development Issues	Fears	Useful Techniques
Infancy (0–1)	Minimal language Feel an extension of parents Sensitive to physical environment	Stranger anxiety	Keep parents in sight Avoid hunger Use warm hands Keep room warm
Toddler (1–3)	Receptive language more advanced than expressive See themselves as individuals Assertive will	Brief separation Pain	Maintain verbal communication Examine with parent when possible Allow some choices when possible
Preschool (3–5)	Excellent expressive skill for thoughts and feelings Rich fantasy life Magical thinking Strong concept of self	Long separation Pain Disfigurement	Allow expression Encourage fantasy and play Encourage participation in care
School age (5–10)	Fully developed language Understanding of body structure and function Able to reason and compromise Experience with self control Incomplete understanding of death	Disfigurement Loss of function Death	Explain procedures Explain pathophysiology and treatment Project positive outcome Stress child's ability to master situation Respect physical modesty
Adolescence (10–19)	Self–determination Decision making Peer group important Realistic view of death	Loss of autonomy Loss of peer acceptance Death	Allow choices and control Stress acceptance by peers Respect autonomy

Table 1.1. Pediatric treatment issues by age group.
Fleisher, Ludwig *Textbook of Pediatric Emergency Medicine,* Copyright Williams & Wilkins 1993.

In infancy, the largest stressor to a child is separation from the parent. Whenever possible, the child should remain in contact with the parent. In addition to providing comfort for the child, the parent can aid in the child's assessment. Parents may assist with the care of their child, but should not be expected to provide health care. Careful reassessment is needed for infants, as it is for adults, to ensure early recognition and management of injuries.

TODDLERS

This stage ranges from 12 to 30 months. These children will be walking and running. They are very inquisitive and make their way into everything. They say words and phrases and may ask for things. They may even follow simple directions. Communication with these children should be in quiet, calming tones. Avoid overly dramatic facial expressions, such as huge grins. Imagine the world from a toddler's point of view, where big scary faces they do not know are yelling instructions at them.

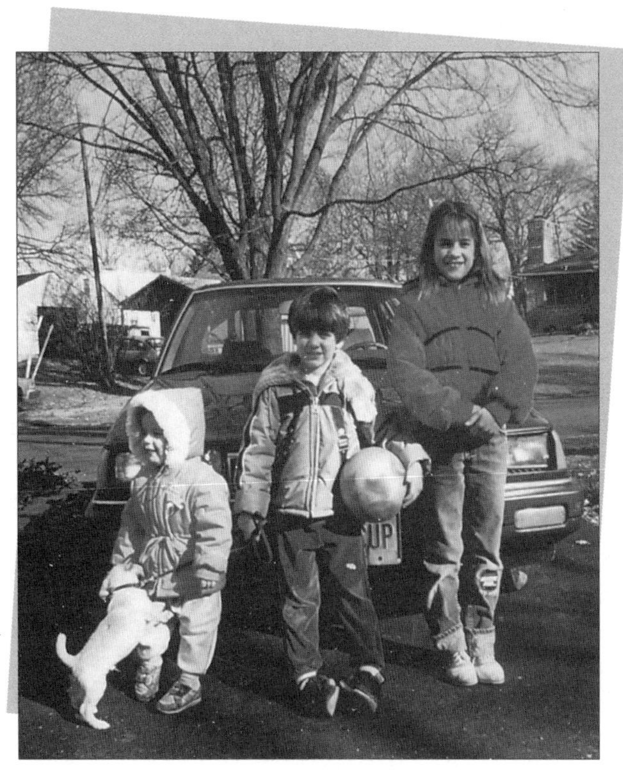

Figure 1.1. Developmental stages.

The greatest stressor to a toddler is parental separation. Special items such as a blanket or toy will be very important to them. Because toddlers have a great fear of restriction of movement, spinal immobilization is quite an ordeal for them. Parental comfort is of utmost importance. These children need to see their parents, hear their voices, or touch them. If the child must be transported, the parent should be allowed to accompany the child to help keep him calm. The parent should be in plain sight of the child; if that is not possible, the parent, at the very least, should be easily heard. Many traumatic injuries can be worsened by increasing the child's stress levels. Parents accompanying children may actually be considered a form of treatment.

Always be honest when performing interventions on these children. Tell them, "This is an ouchie," and "It's okay if you want to cry." Be careful not to say "all done" unless you know for a fact that all painful procedures are done. As a kind gesture to a toddler, the care giver can ask the parent if the child sucks a thumb or fingers and on which hand. Thumb sucking is very popular in this age group; if possible, avoid placing an IV in that hand.

PRESCHOOL

Preschoolers range from age 30 months to 5 years. They can tell you what they want, when they want it, and ask "why?" seemingly a thousand times. These children begin to fear body mutilation. They should be given more preparatory information about what is happening to them and how it will involve their bodies.

Parental involvement is still imperative with this age group. Preschoolers may still have a favorite blanket or toy that would make them more comfortable. As always, honesty is crucial with children and their families, and acceptance of their feelings is very important. Never say to a child, "Why are you crying? It's not that bad."

SCHOOL AGE

School age children range from 6 to 12 years. These children are very good storytellers and historians. They can tell you what is wrong with them and how they were injured. Communication should not be a large problem with this age group because they are beginning to think more concretely and like to talk.

The greatest stressor for these children is loss of bodily control. They need to start making some decisions, when possible, about the care that they receive. If possible, ask them in which hand they would like to have their IV. Are they right handed or left handed? What seems like a small choice to an adult may mean the world to a child.

Parents play a large part in a school–age child's life also. They need to be involved in decision making along with their child. Again, always be honest about procedures. The easiest way to make enemies is to not tell the truth. When in doubt, "I don't know" is the best answer.

ADOLESCENTS

These children range in age from 12 to 18 years. They are notoriously labeled as "difficult" and are fighting to show that they are a valuable part of society. They often have many inner conflicts about whether they want to be treated as a child or an adult. Remember that they are indeed children, but it is imperative that they be involved with their care whenever possible.

The largest stressors to this age group are a lack of trust and enforced dependence. They do not like to think that they are dependent on anyone. Health care will be easier on everyone involved if, when possible, adolescents make decisions about their care. This age group is very particular about parents. Some want their parents with them; others do not. This should be left to them and not be a forced issue.

TRANSPORT CONSIDERATIONS

A stressor that parents often identify is transportation of their children to the hospital. Nothing terrifies parents more than the thought of their child being critically ill or injured, and being transported to the hospital alone and frightened. This is compounded by the fear that the child may not survive the transport to the hospital and that they may not see their child alive again.

If possible, parents should accompany their child to the hospital. Not only are they the best historians regarding their own children, they are also the most welcome source of comfort. Accommodations need to be made for parents to accompany children to the hospital, whether it be by ambulance, helicopter, or fixed–wing aircraft. Good communication is imperative in this situation. Parents must be told what interventions are needed and why. They are not interested in doing a critique on medical care; they are interested in seeing caring people work hard to make their child well again.

Some parents may prefer to follow the emergency vehicle. This may be an acceptable alternative for parents who do not wish to accompany the child. Caution any following vehicles to remain a safe distance from the ambulance and not to follow if lights and sirens will be utilized.

CONFIDENT APPROACH

Although management of pediatric trauma may be difficult for some care givers, a confident, well–organized, systematic approach can be used to evaluate the patient for life-threatening injuries.

The prehospital care giver must be objective, yet understanding, when performing the initial assessment. The key to good patient care is application of the proper assessment technique, knowledge of the disease process, recognition of life–threatening injuries, and initiation of early interventions to increase the chances for a successful outcome.

Even the most difficult case can be managed when an objective approach is used. A chaotic situation can be calmed if the care giver is confident and organized. The team approach to pediatric trauma is essential. The following is an example of an effective prehospital team.

The Team Leader assesses the scene, establishes a rapport with the child and parents, performs initial assessment for life–threatening injuries, makes decisions on patient care guided by the medical control physician or written protocol, and documents the care. This person reports the mechanism of injury, assessment, and interventions to the hospital.

Rescuer 2 stabilizes the c–spine and performs airway maneuvers and management as directed by the in–charge rescuer.

Rescuer 3 selects appropriate equipment and initiates interventions as directed by the in– charge rescuer.

A well–organized team will give every pediatric trauma patient the maximum chance for survival. Every trauma patient, whether an injured bicyclist or an ejected motor vehicle collision victim, must be assessed in the same manner. If assessment is performed in the same way every time, it is less likely that a life–threatening injury will be missed.

EQUIPMENT

Trauma is "no accident" and neither is good patient care. Interventions performed in children, although similar to those performed in adults, are of a different nature and require different techniques.

Children cannot be expanded to fit on or into adult–size equipment, and adult–size equipment cannot be condensed in the field. An applicable medium must be reached. Pediatric–size equipment must be used for the appropriate–size child as much as possible. A variety of manufacturers offer equipment designed especially for children. Child–size airway equipment, cervical immobilization devices, and spinal immobilization equipment are available. When the equipment is not quite suitable, improvisational techniques may be used, ensuring that the objectives of the interventions are met. The skill stations of this book can assist the selection of appropriate equipment.

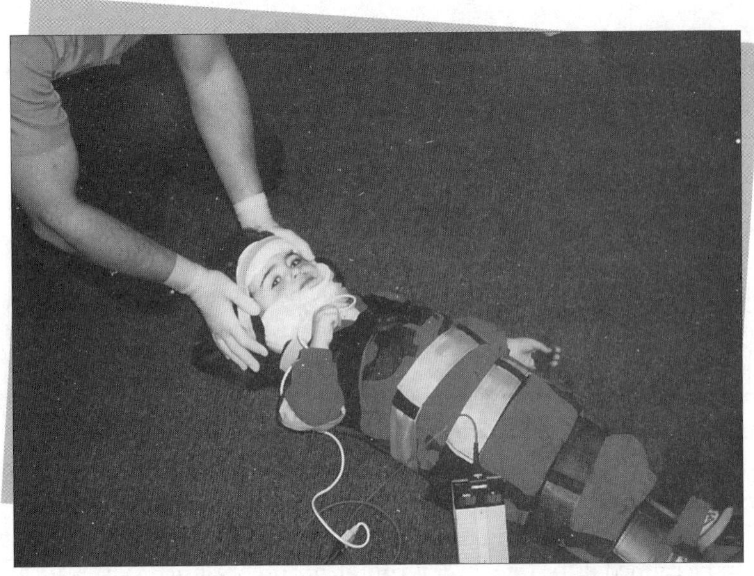

Figure 1.2. A child immobilized with pediatric equipment.

Airway

Bag–valve device and mask sizes # 0,1,2,3
Laryngoscope handle with extra batteries and bulbs
Laryngoscope blades – Straight and/or curved # 0,1,2,3
Stylettes – pediatric
Endotracheal tubes
Uncuffed 2.5–6.0
Cuffed 6.0–8.0
Magill forceps
Water–soluble lubricating jelly
Nasogastric tubes, sizes 5F to 18F
Suction machine and catheters

Vascular Access

Intravenous catheters, sizes 24g to 14g
Intraosseous needles, sizes 16 and 18
Tourniquets, rubber bands
Three–way stop cocks
Syringes
Blood sample tubes
Intravenous tubing, large bore and regular

Intravenous Solutions/Medications

Normal saline or Lactated Ringer's
Atropine
Sodium bicarbonate
Diazepam
Epinephrine
Lidocaine
Naloxone
Pain control medication

Monitoring Equipment

Cardiac monitor/Defibrillator
Pulse oximeter
Glucose analyzer

Immobilization Equipment

Pediatric spinal immobilizer
Cervical collars, pediatric sizes
Cervical immobilization device
Straps to secure patient on board
Pediatric backboard

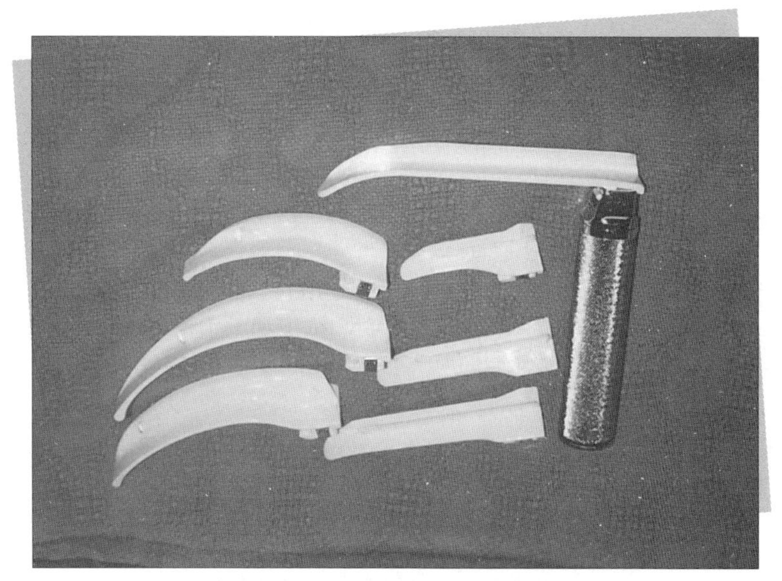

Figure 1.4. Laryngoscope with blades of different sizes.

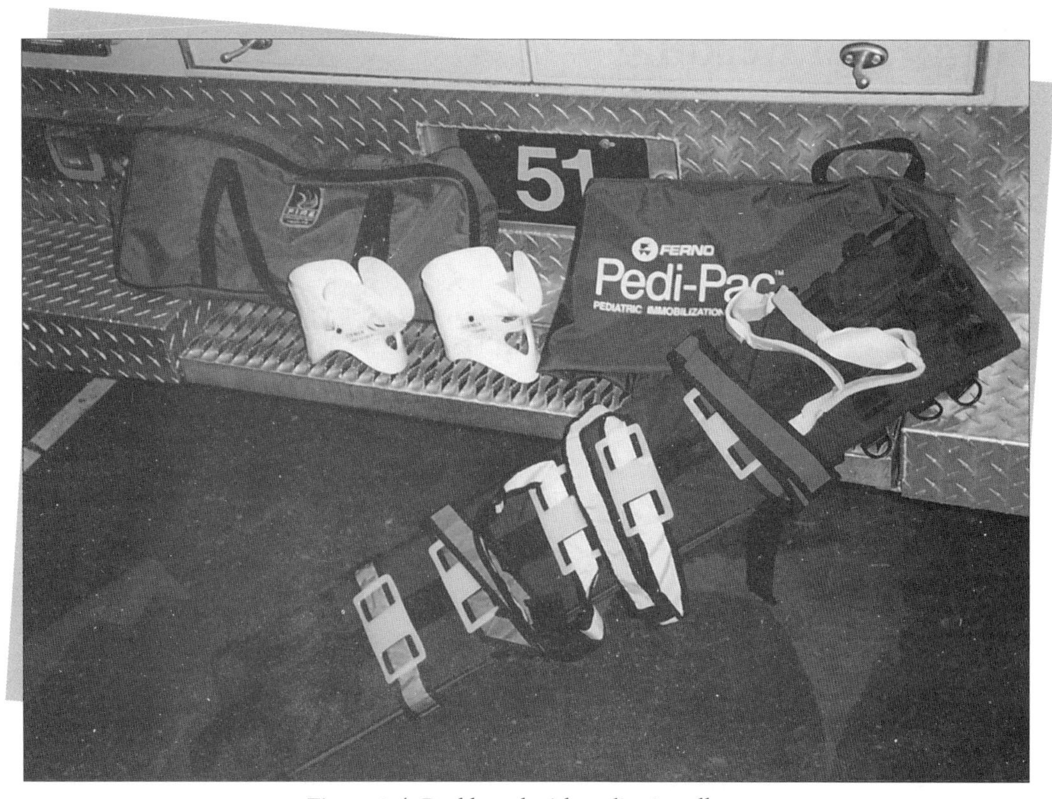

Figure 1.4. Backboard with pediatric collars.

Points to Remember

1. It is essential to communicate with children in a manner that will make assessment easier and more accurate.
2. A well–organized trauma team that practices together and treats every situation in the same way will optimize patient care.
3. In an intense pediatric trauma situation, care givers often panic instead of remembering the basics of trauma care. If care givers apply the techniques described in this book, the injured child will have the best chance for a successful resuscitation.

Bibliography

1. Johnson B, Jeppson E, Redburn L. Caring for children and families: Guidelines for hospitals. *Association for the Care of Childrens Health* 1992;3.
2. Recommended pediatric equipment. American College of Emergency Physicians.

Suggested Reading

1. Brunquell D, Kohen DP. Emotions in pediatric emergencies: What we know, what we can do. *Childrens Health Care* 1991;20(4):240–7.
2. Brown W, Thurman S, Pearce L. Family centered early interventions with infants and toddlers. Innovative cross disciplinary approaches. Paul H. Brooks Publishing, 1993.
3. Johnson K. Trauma in the lives of children. Crisis and stress management for counselors–other professionals. Hunter House Inc., 1989.
4. Thanten, Frankinburg et al. Child health care communications. Enhancing interactions among professionals, parents and children. Johnson and Johnson, 1983.

Common Childhood Injuries

Randy Orsborn, NREMT–P
Sharon Hammond, RN, EMT–A

Introduction

Emergency medical services (EMS) systems are designed primarily for the adult population. Training modalities, equipment design, and overall patient orientation were developed to meet the needs of the ill and injured adult.

Nationally, 5% to 10% of all EMS runs involve pediatric patients. Although children suffer critical injury less frequently than adults (1:10), nearly 50% of all pediatric EMS runs are trauma related.[1–3] Trauma is not simply an adult disease.

Trauma remains the number 1 cause of death and disability for children over the age of 1. Each year trauma kills 22,000 children,[4,5] a large percentage of whom die before reaching the hospital.[1,2] A sizeable number of the survivors suffer significant neurological damage.[1,2] In addition, pediatric injuries account for more than 600,000 hospital admissions and 16 million emergency department visits, for a combined cost of over $7.5 billion.[6] Therefore, EMS providers must take part in community efforts for injury prevention in children.

The problem is evident. Pediatric trauma is a disease process that has reached epidemic proportions. As a prehospital provider, it is essential that, in addition to identifying obvious injuries, you anticipate and identify "hidden" injuries based on how the accident occurred (mechanism of injury).[6–9] This may be accomplished through a quick scene survey on arrival of the EMS unit.

Over the past several decades, the "science" of injury mechanism (also known as the kinetics of trauma)[8,9] has been refined, increasing our awareness of how accidents occur and the injuries that they produce. Numerous texts have addressed the subject, but few have the pediatric victim in mind. This chapter focuses on the mechanisms of pediatric injury by reviewing those mechanisms that occur most frequently, and by addressing common injuries for which effective assessment and treatment modalities have been developed.

TYPE OF TRAUMA

Trauma is generally divided into two categories, blunt and penetrating.

Blunt

Blunt trauma refers to the type of injury resulting from deceleration and/or compression forces (motor vehicle accidents, falls, and sports injuries), which produce internal injury to the underlying tissues. These forces cause compression and/or stretching of the tissue beneath the skin, causing hollow organs (e.g., intestines and stomach) to rupture and spill their contents into the intra–abdominal cavity and solid organs (e.g., liver and spleen) to bleed profusely.

In children, common sites of blunt injury occur at "points of fixation". These are areas where organs or body structures are suspended by ligaments or held in place by bone (Table 2.1).

Organ	Fixation Point
Brain	Cranial nerves and blood vessels
Cervical spine Lumbar spine	Thoracic and sacral spine
Lower trachea	Upper trachea
Descending aorta	Ligamentum arteriosum
Kidneys	Renal vasculature
Liver	Ligamentum teres and hepatic vessels
Urethra	Urogenital diaphragm

Table 2.1. Organs and fixation points.

Penetrating

Penetrating trauma (e.g., stabbings and gunshot wounds) occurs when the skin is broken and the injury extends beneath the open wound. This is usually caused by direct contact with the injury source. Gunshot wounds cause associated tissue injury (i.e., injury to the area around the wound itself) from transmitted energy. This transmission is dependent on the size and type of weapon and speed of the projectile. Penetrating injury is seen more commonly in the urban setting.

MOTOR VEHICLE COLLISION

Motor vehicle collision (MVC)–related trauma accounts for approximately 47% of all pediatric injuries and deaths.[5,10] Contributing factors include failure to use (or improper use of) passenger restraint devices, alcohol use, and adolescent drivers. Half of all adolescent MVC deaths are attributed to alcohol. In younger children, a large number of MVC deaths are attributed to drunk drivers.[5]

An estimated 50% of all pediatric MVC injuries and deaths can be prevented by proper use of child seat and lap–shoulder devices. For children under the age of 4, it is estimated that 70% of their serious injuries and deaths could have been prevented with the use of child restraint devices.[5]

MECHANISM OF INJURY

Examples of MVCs include those involving automobiles, motorcycles, all–terrain vehicles (ATVs), and tractors. The EMS provider must attempt to identify the pathway of injury to the occupants by first observing the mode of transportation. Predictable injury patterns are best recognized by maintaining a high index of suspicion.

For example, if the child was involved in a collision, the rescuer should attempt to obtain as much information about the accident as possible. Visual inspection of the vehicle may help reveal both expected and unexpected injuries. Damage to the vehicle is an indicator of the forces involved. Deformity of the interior of the vehicle helps to indicate the child's impact, based on where the child was positioned, and clues to possible injuries. In other words, the extent of damage to the vehicle relates to the extent of injury to the child.

Observe for restraint devices. Most automobile manufacturers have restraint devices designed for the adult passenger. One recent study has demonstrated that approximately 60% of the U.S. population uses auto safety restraint devices improperly. Unused or improperly positioned restraints may subject the child to additional injury during the accident. If the infant is correctly restrained in a car seat, but the car seat is not properly restrained, the child may be ejected from the car or strike various structures in the car. Note if the car seat is found still restrained. Although a child may have been restrained properly, the care giver should maintain a high index of suspicion because the child may have sustained serious injuries. Seat belts, when improperly used, may also cause injuries to the abdomen and the lumbar spine of a child (Chapter 7).

Pediatric MVC victims often appear unharmed. However, it is important to watch for hidden injury. Impact with the windshield may produce obvious head and facial injuries, but the rescuer should suspect the need for airway intervention and spinal immobilization for possible spinal trauma.

Chest injuries such as flail chest, myocardial contusion, pulmonary contusion, simple and tension pneumothoraces, and great–vessel trauma should be assessed if the child struck the dash, rear of the front seat, or other object inside the vehicle.

Ejection from the motor vehicle accounts for approximately 27% of all vehicular deaths. Impact with the ground, a tree, or other fixed object increases the child's risk for significant c–spine injury. Partial ejection carries an increased risk of extremity trauma.

PEDESTRIAN INJURIES

Children ages 5 to 9 are at the greatest risk of being struck and killed by a motor vehicle.[6–9] Injuries commonly occur when a child runs out into the street. Because children are easily distracted and lack quick reflexive action, they often are injured while chasing a toy, friend, or pet into the path of an oncoming vehicle.

In the United States (and other countries where automobiles are driven on the right side of the road), the vehicle first strikes the left side of the child. The bumper contacts the left femur, and the fender strikes the left side of the abdomen. The child then is thrown against the hood or windshield of the vehicle. As the automobile comes to a halt, the child is thrown to the ground, striking the head on the pavement. This bumper–hood–ground mechanism of injury is referred to as Waddell's Triad (Figure 2.1) and often produces femur, spleen, and head injuries. The child then is often run over by the vehicle. The rescuer should maintain a high degree of suspicion for this combination of injuries when evaluating a child who has been struck by a motor vehicle.

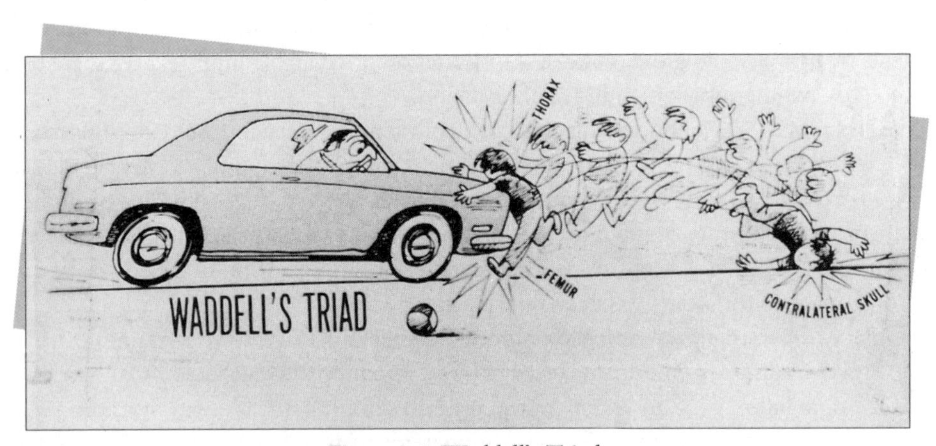

Figure 2.1. Waddell's Triad.

BICYCLE INJURIES

There are more than 100 million bicyclists in the United States. Bicycle collisions account for an estimated 200,000 injuries and over 600 deaths to children each year.[5] Approximately 80% of all childhood bicycling accidents occur on residential streets within five blocks of home.[11] Most bicycle riders involved in accidents have less than one year of riding experience.[11]

Collisions between motor vehicles and bicycles are commonly associated with children who are in violation of a traffic law (e.g., riding on the wrong side of the road and riding into traffic from alleys, side streets, driveways, etc.). In children younger than 12, deaths occur when the victim was struck from the left, after riding in front of an oncoming vehicle. Older children tend to be struck from behind.[11]

Head trauma is the leading cause of injury and death in most bicycle–related accidents. One recent study depicting the frequency of head injuries in bicycle–collisions victims revealed that 69% of these patients suffered head injuries. Twenty–three percent suffered orthopedic injuries, and 25% were admitted for soft–tissue injuries and lacerations (the overlap was attributed to victims with multiple–system injury).[12]

Because the child's head is relatively large in relation to the rest of the body (25% of body weight), he is more likely to suffer significant head trauma. For this reason, the rescuer should anticipate that there is serious injury to the head and direct resuscitation efforts accordingly. (Remember, an injury above the clavicle area is considered to be a c–spine injury until proven otherwise.)

Bicycle helmets can prevent an estimated 85% of head trauma and 88% of brain injuries.[5,11] Because many parents are unaware of the need for helmets, attempts to increase bicycle helmet usage should be made through public education. Children, family members, and health care providers need to be educated continually on helmet availability and the advantages of helmet use.

FALLS

Falls are the single most common cause of injury in the pediatric population and account for approximately one–third of all trauma admissions.[14] These children tend to be younger, less than 3 years old, and playing at the time of injury.[4,14] Fortunately, the mortality rate is low (0.7%) but morbidity is high, with over 60% of the children sustaining a fracture and a number left neurologically impaired from a head injury.[10] Important factors to consider in a fall are the height from which the child fell, the mass of the child, and the surface the child contacted. If the child fell onto a wet grass surface, the probability of serious injury is much lower than if he contacted cement. Care givers should note the way the child landed and on what part of the body.

In urban areas, falls account for a significant number of serious injuries, particularly head trauma. In New York City, falls resulted in 20% of all unintentional traumatic deaths.[4,14] Following a simple epidemiologic study, which demonstrated a clear relationship between warm weather and falls from windows, the city undertook a program to install window guards in apartments housing young children. Deaths caused by falls decreased markedly following the institution of this program. Other areas of the country have identified the serious morbidity that may result from falls, particularly in younger children, and are in the process of developing injury prevention strategies.

FIREARMS

Firearms, handguns in particular, produce the most common form of penetrating injury in the "civilized" world. Gunshot wounds are the sixth leading cause of accidental death in the United States.[10] In fact, the United States has the highest firearm–related homicide rate of any nation, more than four times that of any other country.[4,5,10]

Fifty percent of all American homes have firearms, with one in four having a handgun.[5] In a recent study, 34% of all high school students indicated that they could easily obtain a gun.[5] Students are frequently carrying guns to school. When evaluating the mechanism of firearm–related injury, the care giver should note, if possible, whether the injury was from an accidental (unintentional) versus an intentional cause. This determination usually has a direct relationship to the scene itself. For example, the majority of unintentional shootings occur at home. The shooting may have been the result of a curious child at the wrong end of the weapon. The availability of the gun at home has also been linked to an increase in adolescent suicide.

When evaluating the mechanism of injury of penetrating trauma, wound ballistics must be taken into consideration. Trajectory of the object, the energy dissipation, and the type of projectile will influence injury severity.[13] Table 2.2 lists physical findings of common firearm–related injuries.

Body Area	Physical Findings
Head	Facial and skull areas (in attempted suicide) Excessive bleeding Airway obstruction from bleeding
Neck	Excessive hemorrhage from large (major) vessel Airway dysfunction C–spine injury
Chest	Lungs (pulmonary contusion/open pneumothorax) Heart (tamponade, empty–heart syndrome) Ribs (fractures/flail segments)
Abdomen	Contusion/massive bleeding Hollow–organ rupture
Extremities	Bleeding/fracture Vascular compromise

Table 2.2. Common firearm–related injuries.

Points to Remember

1. Millions of children are victims of trauma in our society. The four most common forms of childhood accidents are MVCs, pedestrian injuries, bicycle accidents, and gunshot wounds.
2. When assessing these children, remember that many of their injuries will be obvious; some will not be obvious. The mechanism of injury serves as a guide to help recognize the hidden, less–obvious injuries.
3. Trauma is the leading cause of death and disability in children over the age of 1; in addition, the care required is very expensive. Fortunately, in most cases, trauma is preventable. EMS providers must take an active part in not only the treatment of pediatric trauma, but in its prevention.

Bibliography

1. Cooper A, Barlow B, Davidson L, et al: Epidemiology of pediatric trauma: Importance of popular–based statistics. *J Pediatr Surg* 1989;27:149.
2. Oreskovich M: Prehospital surgical care, in Mayer TA: *Transportation of the Injured Child.*
3. Foltin GL, Tunik, MG: Emergency medical services for children in Barkin RM (ed): *Pediatric Emergency Medicine: Concepts and Clinical Practice.* St Louis, Mosby–Yearbook, 1992.
4. Peclet MH, Newman KD, et al: Patterns of injury in children. *J Pediatr Surg* 1990; 25: 85– 91.
5. Lundberg GD (ed): Pediatric basic life support. *JAMA* 1992;268:2251–2252.
6. Campbell JE: *Basic Trauma Life Support.* Englewood Cliffs, New Jersey, Brady Co, 1988.
7. McSwain NE: *Kinematics of Blunt Injury.* Akron, Ohio, Emergency Training,1984.
8. Stewart C: *Mechanisms of injury.* Emergency Medical Sevices, 1989.
9. Butman AM, Paturas JL: *Prehospital Trauma Life Support.* Akron, Ohio. Emergency Training, 1986.
10. Division of Injury Control Center for Environmental Health and Injury Control, Centers for Disease Control: Childhood injuries in the United States. *Am J Dis Child* 1990;144:627–646.
11. Storo W: The role of bicycle helmets in bicycle–related injury prevention. *Clin Pediatr* 1992; July:421– 427.
12. Lundberg GO (ed): Special resuscitation situations. *JAMA* 1992;268:2242–2250.
13. Gallaher MM, Fleming DW, et al: Pedestrian and hypothermic deaths among Native Americans in New Mexico: Between bar and home. *JAMA* 1992;267:1345–1348.
14. Fackler M: Ballistic injury. Ann Emerg Med 1986;15:1451–1455.
15. Lehman D, Schonfeld N: Falls from heights: A problem not just in the Northeast. *Pediatrics* 1993;92:121–124.

Assessment of the Pediatric Trauma Patient

Ann M.Dietrich, MD
Steven J. Shaner, EMT–P

Introduction

Trauma is the leading cause of death among children over the age of one year, with most of the mortality resulting from multiple trauma. Although children can have a multitude of serious injuries, most medical personnel are inexperienced in the management of these younger patients. A standard, organized approach ensures the appropriate management of multiply injured, unstable pediatric patients.

The assessment of children and adults is similar, but the physiologic response of a child to trauma is different. The most important thing to do prior to arrival at the scene is to correctly prepare the equipment that will be needed. The appropriate–size equipment should be easily accessible. If the parents are at the scene, present yourself in a very organized, efficient manner and use them as a resource.

When a patient is stable, involve the parents as much as possible in the care of their child. Various age groups respond differently, as is explained in greater detail in Chapter 1. If the child is critically injured, obtain a very brief history and explain to the parents how important rapid package and transport can be for an injured child. Move quickly to the child and begin a rapid assessment.

Because children vary in size, a precalculated tape (i.e. Broselow® Tape) may be used to estimate weight and appropriate–size equipment. Normal vital signs for different age groups are shown in Table 3.1. Do not trust your memory; carry a card that has the normal values for age listed on it.

Age	Weight in kg (lb)	Respirations	Pulse	Systolic Blood Pressure
Newborn	3–4 kg (6–9 lb)	30–50	120–160	60–80
6 mo–1 yr	8–10 kg (16–22 lb)	30–40	120–140	70–80
2–4 yr	12–16 kg (24–34 lb)	20–30	100–110	80–95
5–8 yr	18–26 kg (36–55 lb)	14–20	90–100	90–100
8–12 yr	26–50 kg (55–110 lb)	12–20	80–100	100–110
>12 yr	>50 kg (110 lb)	12–16	60–90	100–120

Table 3.1. Weight and vital signs by age group.

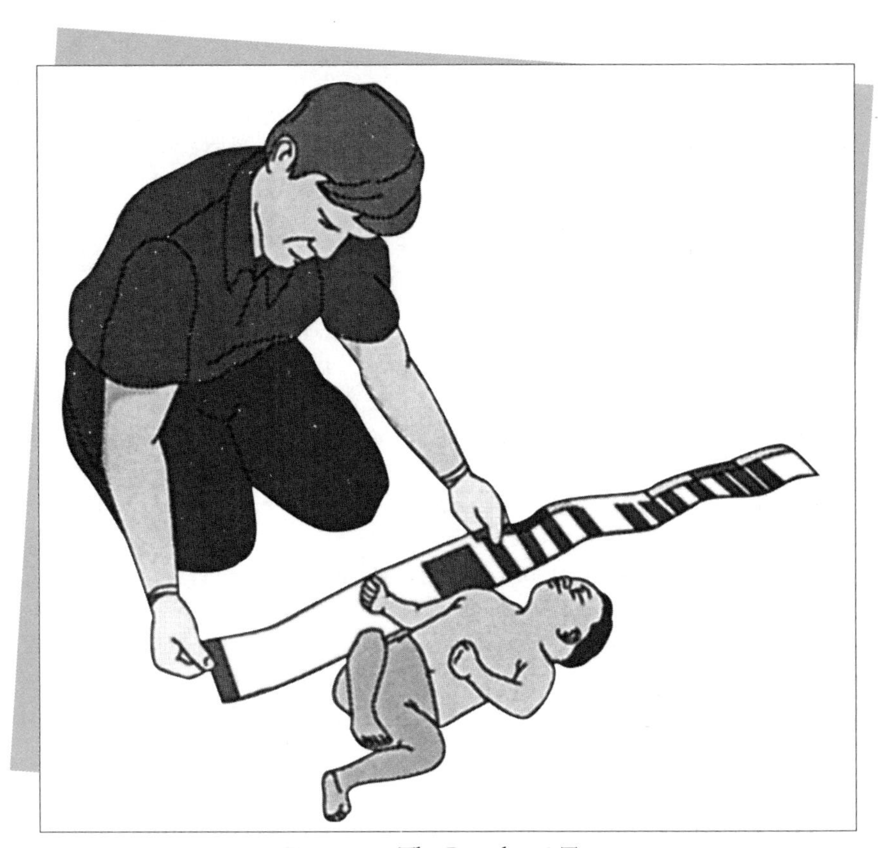

Figure 3.1. The Broselow ® Tape.

ASSESSMENT

The most common ways children get injured are motor vehicle crashes, as pedestrians or bicycle riders struck by a car, falls, abuse, burns, and drowning. As indicated in Chapter 2, always consider the mechanism in relation to the size of the child. In general, the following approach should be used:

1. Scene survey
2. Airway, c–spine control, and initial LOC
3. Breathing
4. Circulation
5. Brief exam of abdomen, pelvis, and extremities
6. Critical transport decisions
7. Package and transport interventions
8. Secondary survey

Scene Survey

The scene should be assessed for mechanism of injury, safety, and other victims.

During the primary trauma survey, all critical injuries should be identified and a decision made regarding the need for urgent transport. The primary trauma survey should be completed in 2 minutes or less. *The primary trauma survey should not be interrupted except for an obstructed airway or a cardiopulmonary arrest. The primary trauma survey consists of a scene survey, evaluation of the child's airway with c–spine control, breathing, circulation, and brief examination of the abdomen, pelvis and extremities.*

Airway and C–spine

The first few seconds of evaluation reveal valuable information. Is the child looking at you? Does he recognize his parents? While assessing the airway, it is imperative that the c–spine be manually maintained. In children, the head is relatively large compared to the rest of the body, so make sure the neck is immobilized in a neutral position. *Always assume the child's neck is injured and maintain c–spine precautions throughout the assessment and management of the patient.*

As the neck is stabilized, assess the airway. Although a screaming child may be difficult to deal with, screaming usually means an open airway. Recognize the signs of upper airway occlusion, apnea, stridor, and agonal respirations. Listen carefully for air movement through the mouth. If the child is unconscious, open the airway using the modified jaw thrust maneuver. Listen carefully again. Children have a tendency to produce more secretions than adults. Have suction available and use it to clear the mouth of any blood or secretions. If an assistant is available, have this person place oxygen on the patient. *Always administer 100% oxygen.*

Breathing

Following the stabilization of the airway, the child's breathing must be assessed. Look at the patient's respiratory rate, oxygenation, and efforts to breathe. Compare the respiratory rate of the child to the normal rate listed on the card for the age of the child.

Initially, when children are in respiratory distress they breathe very quickly (tachypnea). As they have more problems breathing, the respiratory rate slows and periods of apnea may occur. Look at the color of the child's lips and nail beds. They should be pink. If they're not, the child may be hypoxic. Observe how hard the child is working to breathe. Note nostril flaring, retractions, and grunting. Look for the position of the trachea and venous distention. Listen carefully to the child's lung fields; assess how well they are moving air.

If the child is apneic or having severe respiratory distress, initiate ventilatory assistance. A second rescuer should give 100% oxygen via an appropriately sized mask; while maintaining a good seal, ventilate at the rate the child would normally breathe. If the child has been apneic or has a head injury, hyperventilate until a CO_2 measuring device is obtained (this most likely will be at the hospital). Hyperventilate at a rate that is eight to ten ventilations per minute faster than the child would normally breathe. Watch the chest for rise and fall and listen carefully to the lungs for air exchange. It is preferable not to intubate the child in the field. Intubation is often time–consuming and technically difficult in the pediatric patient. If the child can be effectively oxygenated and ventilated with a bag–valve–mask, do not use precious time attempting intubation prior to transport. Maintain the child's airway with bag–valve–mask ventilations and remember to keep suction available for management of secretions.

If the child has evidence of a tension pneumothorax, as described in Chapter 5, this problem must be corrected rapidly or the child may progress to cardiopulmonary arrest. Treatment involves needle decompression performed in the manner described in Skill Station 2.

Circulation

Next, the circulation of the child must be evaluated. Note the pulse. A well–perfused child should have a strong peripheral pulse (radial or dorsalis pedis). If this is absent, check for a central pulse (brachial, femoral, or carotid). Count the pulse and check your card to see if this is normal for age or too fast or too slow. The best indicators of shock in a child will be tachycardia, weak peripheral pulses, and prolonged capillary refill. Infants sometimes will appear mottled. This may be a sign of poor perfusion or a result of being cold or scared.

Blood pressure is helpful but is usually very difficult to obtain in the field. If there is time and you have the appropriate equipment, a blood pressure reading may be obtained en route to the hospital; however, do not waste time, particularly in a severely injured child. *Remember that hypotension is a late finding in shock.* Immediate actions should include stopping all obvious bleeding and ensuring that the child is kept as warm as possible.

Examine the Abdomen, Pelvis, and Extremities (Quick Survey)

Prior to placing the child on the backboard, rapidly expose and look at the child's abdomen. Gently palpate all four abdominal quadrants and note any contusions, abrasions, penetrations, or distention. If there is no complaint of pain in the pelvic area, palpate the pelvis noting any tenderness, instability, or crepitus. The lower extremities should be quickly evaluated for deformity, contusions, abrasions, penetrations, burns, tenderness, lacerations, or swelling.

Brief Neurologic Assessment

By this time, a brief neurologic examination has been completed by observation of the child. It has been noted whether the child is alert (A), responding to verbal commands (V), responding only to pain (P), or is unresponsive (U). See Chapter 8 for the modified Glasgow Coma Scale for children.

Continue to observe the child the entire time he is being packaged for transport. Children with severe head injuries will usually be very sleepy and not respond appropriately to you or their parents. If the child is unresponsive, the airway must be secured with bag–valve–mask ventilations or intubation. Remember to hyperventilate all children suspected of having a head injury.

By this time, the child should be adequately exposed to assess all the injuries. *You can't assess what you can't see!* Remember to log roll the child the same way as an adult and to check the patient's back carefully for any injuries.

Critical Transport Decisions

Children with any of the following problems should be packaged and transported as quickly as possible to a pediatric center:

1. Unstable airway
2. Obvious respiratory insufficiency
3. Shock
4. Altered mental status

In these situations, *rapid* transport is critical. The decision over mode of transport should be guided by local protocols that take into account the acuity of the illness and the time to the receiving hospital. Situations in which early arrival at a pediatric center may make a significant difference in outcome include cold–water drowning, critical airways, shock, severe head injuries, and multiple injuries.

Package and Transport Interventions

Airway and C–spine. Maintain c–spine control during the packaging process. If an appropriate–size rigid collar is available, place it on the patient and secure the collar and the patient to the backboard. If an appropriate collar is not available, secure the patient to the board in the neutral position. C–spine immobilization may be difficult, especially in the young child, as will be addressed in Chapter 7 and Skill Station 1.

If bag–valve–mask ventilation is effective, intubation may be deferred until the patient is at the hospital. If the child requires intubation, it should be performed en route to the receiving facility. *C–spine control must always be maintained.* If the child requires intubation, make sure the endotracheal tube is well secured in the correct position. Listen carefully to the breath sounds after placement. Note the rise and fall of the chest; these should be symmetric. Check the mucous membranes and nail beds for oxygenation. Pulse oximetry, if available, will also help in assessing how well oxygen is moving through the body. The goal should be to keep the oxygen saturation as close to 100% as possible.

Breathing. Airway and breathing are very closely tied together. Once the airway is secured, the child's ventilation should be assessed. If the patient is intubated, be sure the tube is in the correct position. Use the items stressed in Chapter 4 to confirm tube placement: condensation, auscultation, and compliance. If available, pulse oximetry and capnography can assist in verifying that the endotracheal tube is in the correct position.

Use the assessment described in Chapter 5 (tracheal position, auscultation, and compliance) to identify chest injuries. All patients should have oxygen saturation readings of 100%. If the child's condition changes at any time, perform the reassessment survey.

Circulation. Early recognition and management of shock are critical. Even if the child has no airway or breathing difficulties, he should be placed on 100% oxygen. This will maximize the oxygen delivery to the poorly perfused tissues.

Use of the pneumatic antishock device is controversial. If the child is over 6 years old (weighs over 25 to 35 kg), the leg components may be utilized. Inflation of the abdominal compartment is a relative contraindication because it may cause compression of the chest cavity and difficulty with breathing. Pneumatic antishock trousers should not be used in children with isolated severe head injuries, or penetrating chest and abdominal wounds. As in adults, an assessment of the lower extremities should be completed prior to their application.

IV access may be obtained en route, but if a prolonged extrication is required, it can be obtained at the scene. IV access may be difficult, especially if the patient has multisystem injury and is in shock. If IV access is obtained, 20 mL/kg of lactated Ringer's should be given as a fluid bolus. Recheck heart rate, pulses, and perfusion after every bolus to evaluate progress. As soon as the heart rate and perfusion have returned to normal, IV fluids should be run at keep–open rates. This will prevent the child from becoming fluid overloaded. If local protocols allow, intraosseous infusions may be used for the treatment of critically injured children. Do not attempt an intraosseous line unless the patients airway and respiratory status have been stabilized (Skill Station 3).

When you arrive at the hospital, advise the trauma team of the total amount of fluids the child has received.

Secondary Survey

The secondary survey is a detailed examination of the patient from head to toe. The acuity of the injuries and the time available prior to your arrival at the receiving institution will determine how much of this will be completed.

Remember that the primary trauma survey should be the first priority! In general, a critical patient should have the secondary survey completed en route to the hospital, and a stable child should have it performed at the scene. Early recognition and management of the ABCs is critical!!

Head assessment. A complete examination of the head, noting cuts, bruises, hematomas, and depressions is important. If the child has an open fontanelle, note whether it is flat or bulging. Note any fluid or blood from the nose and ears (basilar skull fracture). Check the pupils and note whether they are equal and whether they react to light.

Neck examination. Note the external appearance of the neck. Note the position of the trachea and if the neck veins are distended or flat. Often this will be difficult in the young child or infant because the neck is short, fat, and difficult to assess.

Thoracic examination. Watch the chest rise and fall. Note symmetry and any bruises or crepitus. Listen carefully to the breath sounds.

Abdominal examination. Note any abdominal bruises or marks (e.g., seat belt). Also note if the patient has abdominal distention, tenderness, or guarding. Note pelvic stability.

Extremity examination. Note the location of any deformities and check the neurovascular status below the site of the injury. All active sites of bleeding should have been stopped during the primary survey, but make sure the dressings are securely in place for transport. Carefully package any amputated parts.

Neurologic examination. Complete the neurologic examination at this point. Make sure the child is moving all extremities and has good muscle strength. Again, recheck the pupils.

PACKAGING FOR TRANSPORT

Even if the child is severely injured, it is important to make sure that he is appropriately immobilized prior to transport. Place the correct size c–collar and secure the child to the backboard. Always be sure to secure the body to the backboard first and then the child's head. C–spine control can be maintained only when both the head and the body are immobilized. Make sure all tubes are secured, especially endotracheal tubes and gastric tubes. Place the monitor leads on the child and monitor during transport.

Sample History

While packaging the child, obtain as much history from the patient, parents, and family as possible. A "sample" history contains the following information:

S Symptoms

A Allergies, particularly medications and immunization status

M Medications the child is on or the parents have given

P Past illnesses, particularly bleeding disorders, congenital problems, heart disease, and birth history

L Last meal. Make a note of what the child had and what time it was

E Events preceding the injury

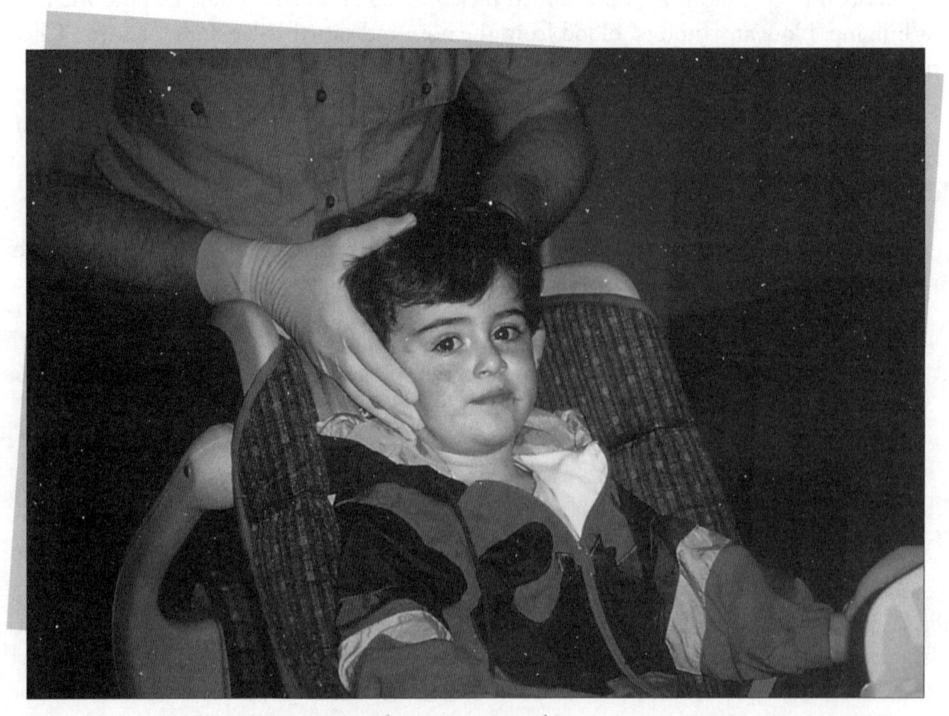

Figure 3.2. Manual c–spine control in a trauma patient.

REASSESSMENT SURVEY

1. Recheck level of consciousness and pupils
2. Reassess ABCs
3. Recheck abdomen
4. Focused assessment of injuries
5. Check interventions

Points to Remember

1. Always consider the mechanism of injury and the size of the child. Prepare the correct equipment prior to arrival at the scene if possible.
2. Stick with the basics – c–spine control, airway, breathing, and circulation. Reassess the child continually.
3. If the child's condition changes, go back to the basics! Ensure an adequate airway, a stable respiratory status, and adequate circulation.
4. Make sure that you continue to assess and reassess the patient!
5. *Rapid assessment, appropriate interventions, and transport to an appropriate facility are the key ingredients to long–term patient survival. You make the difference!*

The Pediatric Airway

Ann M. Dietrich, MD

Introduction

The respiratory system delivers oxygen to the blood and eliminates carbon dioxide. Inadequate function of this system, respiratory distress, in an infant or a child may rapidly progress to respiratory failure and finally to cardiopulmonary arrest. Respiratory compromise is a leading cause of prehospital arrests, with most children having a poor outcome once a cardiac arrest has occurred. Early management of the child's airway following a traumatic event is critical to allow for adequate oxygenation and ventilation. *In children, early recognition and management of an airway problem are crucial.*

ANATOMY/PHYSIOLOGY

The pediatric airway differs from the adult airway in many important ways. Anatomic differences of the upper airway include the following: the tongue is relatively larger in proportion to the rest of the oral cavity; the larynx is higher in the neck (C3–4) compared with that of the adult (C4–5); the infant epiglottis is angled away from the long axis of the trachea; the vocal folds are attached anteriorly at a lower level than posteriorly; and the subglottic area is the narrowest portion of the infant larynx (Figure 4.1).

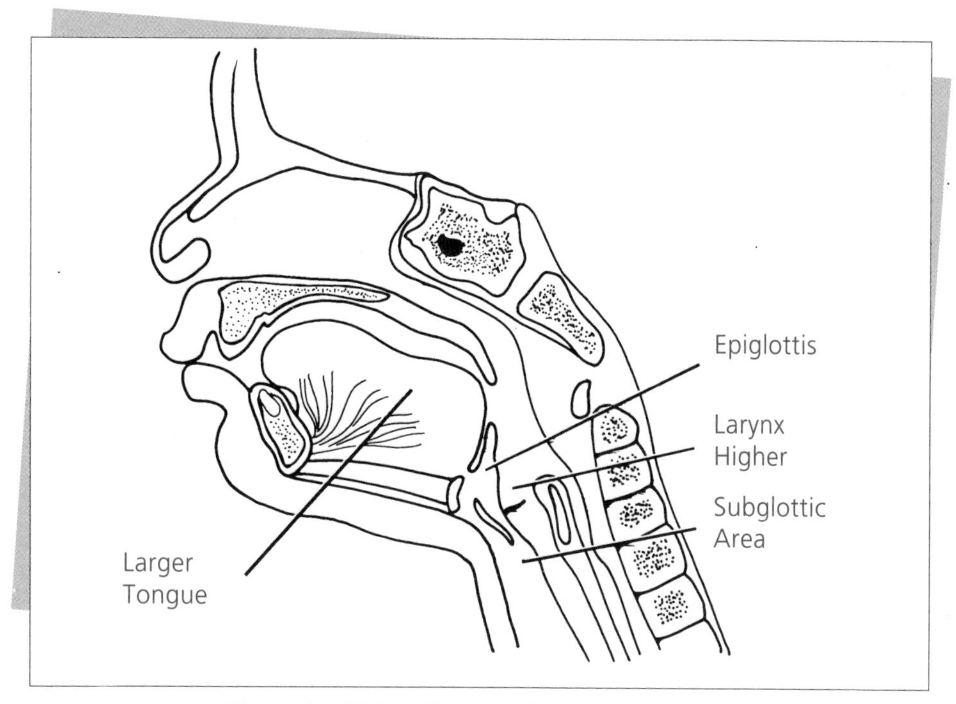

Figure 4.1. Unique features of the pediatric airway.

The airways of children are smaller, and the supporting cartilage is less developed. Because of their smaller size, they can be easily obstructed by mucus, blood, or edema. Airway obstruction results in increased resistance (Figure 4.2).

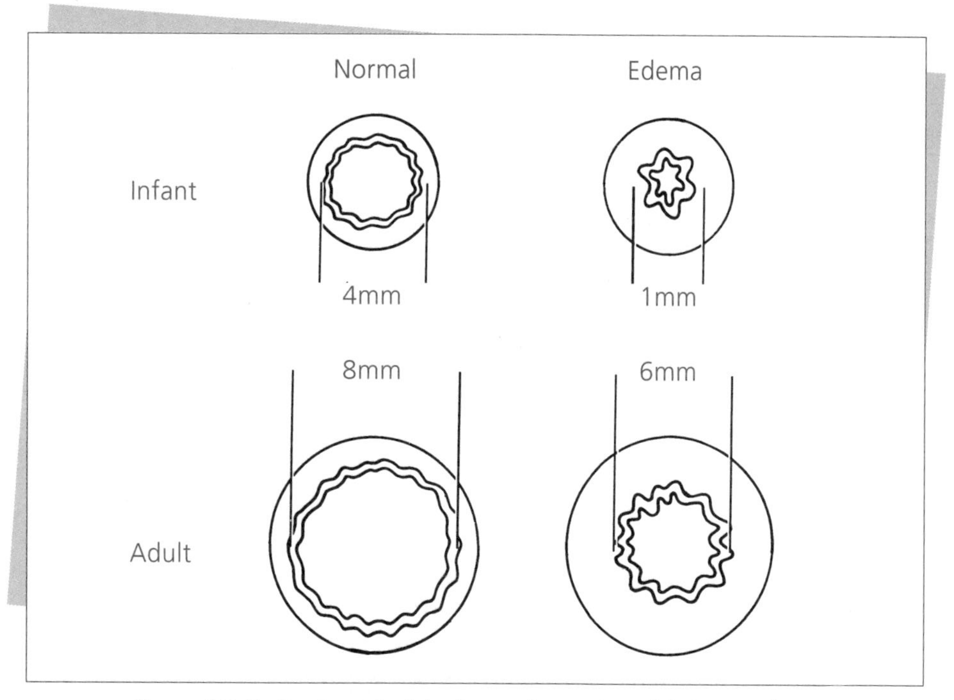

Figure 4.2. Pediatric and adult airway obstruction with 1 mm edema.

Mechanically, children have problems compensating for respiratory difficulties. In young children, the ribs are very pliable and fail to support the lungs. This may lead to paradoxical movement of the chest (sternal and intercostal retractions) when respiratory difficulty occurs. Because children have poorly developed muscles and less compensatory reserve than adults, the progression from respiratory distress to respiratory failure may occur quickly. In addition, the child's tidal volume is dependent on diaphragmatic function and movement. Therefore, gastric or abdominal distention may impede effective respirations. The pediatric patient is further compromised by a high metabolic rate (oxygen consumption is 6 to 8 mL/kg/min in a child compared to 3 to 4 mL/kg/min in an adult). When inadequate respirations or apnea occur, hypoxemia will develop rapidly.

Other conditions, such as hypothermia, overdoses, metabolic derangements, and head trauma, may also result in airway compromise or aggravate an already compromised airway.

The goal of emergency airway therapy is early recognition and rapid intervention.

ASSESSMENT

Airway assessment is the most critical aspect of care for a pediatric trauma victim. Failure to identify an airway problem in a child may lead to further patient compromise and cardiopulmonary arrest. *Maintaining an open airway is critical.*

The patient assessment sequence places airway assessment after a quick scene assessment.

1. Scene survey
2. Airway, c–spine control, and initial LOC
3. Breathing
4. Circulation
5. Brief exam of abdomen, pelvis, and extremities
6. Critical transport decisions
7. Package and transport interventions
8. Secondary survey

Scene Survey

The scene survey should be handled as taught in BTLS. Establish the safety of the environment and gain as much information as possible regarding the mechanism of injury to aid with the child's assessment and stabilization. Carefully evaluate the scene for evidence of fire and damage to the vehicle. Whenever possible, note restraining devices used and how the child was positioned in them. Placing small children in adult restraining devices may result in an injury. For example, a shoulder strap that crosses the child's trachea may cause injury to that area.

Airway and C–spine

As described Chapter 3, all pediatric trauma patients should have their cervical spines immobilized. As manual control of the neck is taken, determine whether the child has an open airway.

If the child is not breathing or is making obstructive airway noises, open the airway with a modified jaw thrust maneuver. If the airway is obstructed, think of a foreign body; children are always placing things in their mouths. Reposition again and begin bag–valve–mask ventilations. If a single provider is having difficulty providing effective bag–valve–mask ventilations, a second provider may assist the first provider. Always use 100% oxygen and make sure that there is chest movement with each administered breath. The volume of each ventilation should be 10 mL/kg. So, a 20–kg child should receive 200 mL of tidal volume per breath. As shown in Skill Station 2, mask size should be based on achieving a tight seal over the face with the mask extending from the bridge of the nose to the cleft of the chin.

An oropharyngeal airway may be inserted in an unconscious child to assist with maintaining an open airway. If a child cannot be ventilated with a bag–valve–mask, the child should be intubated using in–line c–spine stabilization.

In children with a complete obstruction of the upper airway due to foreign body, severe oropharyngeal injuries, or a laryngeal fracture, a cricothyroidotomy may be required. However, this procedure is contraindicated in children under 12 years old. Although most airways can be opened with airway manipulations, this procedure may be life–saving when indicated. The technique is discussed in Skill Station 2.

Breathing

If the child is breathing, determine the effectiveness of the respirations. One sign of an upper airway obstruction is stridor, an inspiratory high–pitched sound, which may be caused by a congenital abnormality, foreign body, or infection. In a trauma situation involving a previously normal child, stridor is usually caused by a foreign body, laryngeal injury, or upper airway swelling. If the child is adequately maintaining his airway, immobilize and transport. Any visible foreign objects should be removed. Most children will have a patent airway when the head is placed in a neutral position (Fig 4.3).

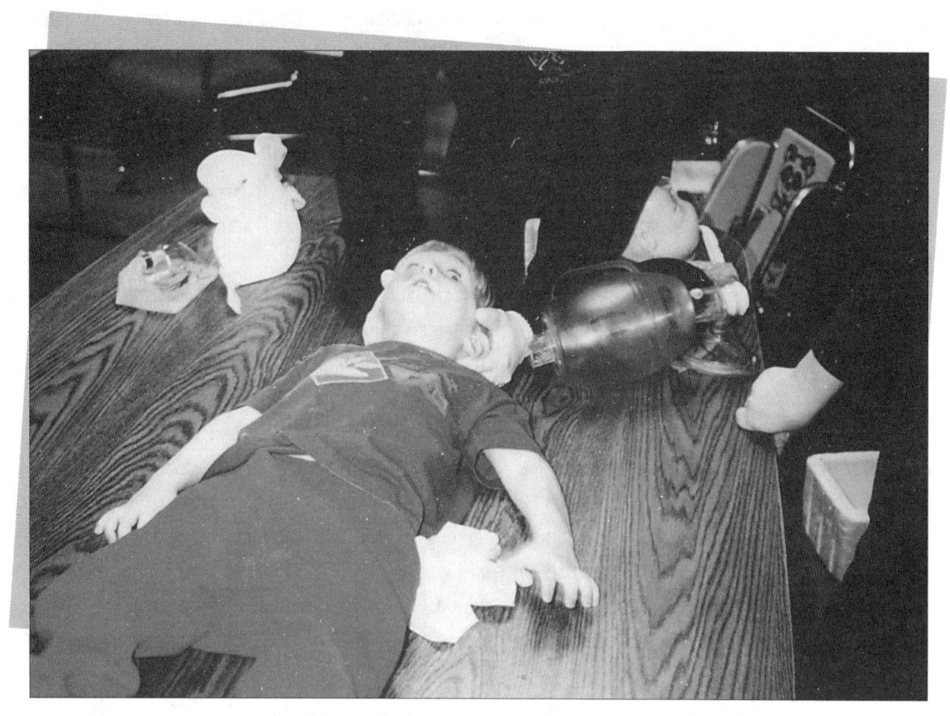

Figure 4.3. Neutral position with manual c–spine control.

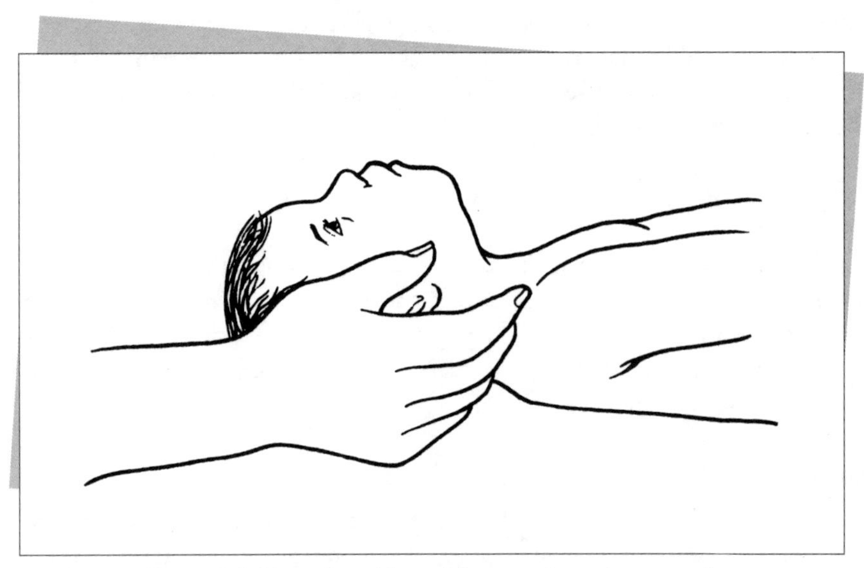

Figure 4.3. Neutral position with manual c–spine control.

When assessing pediatric breath sounds, it is important to listen to both lung fields and to determine the child's "work" of breathing. Because children have such a thin chest wall, breath sounds are easily transmitted and may be misleading. For example, in children with a pneumothorax, the breath sounds may not be absent. Wheezing or a prolonged expiratory phase may be present if the child has aspirated or has a preexisting problem with asthma. Whether the respiratory problem involves the upper airway or the lower airway, care givers must decide if the child's oxygenation and ventilation are adequate. Signs of respiratory distress include tachypnea (fast breathing), nasal flaring, retractions, and grunting.

First assess the child's respiratory rate and compare it with the normal respiratory rate for that age (Table 3.1). Increased work of breathing is shown by nasal flaring and retractions. Retractions involve the child's use of accessory muscles, intercostal, subcostal, and suprasternal, to assist with adequate oxygen delivery and ventilation. Grunting is a sound produced by premature glottic closure accompanying chest wall contraction. This is the child's attempt to increase airway pressure and keep the airway open. *When a child is showing signs of respiratory distress, it is very important to determine the etiology and plan intervention to prevent the progression to respiratory failure.* All children with evidence of respiratory distress should receive 100% oxygen. The airway should be assessed to be sure it is open, and the chest should be assessed for evidence of a pneumothorax, hemothorax, or bony injury (i.e., rib fracture).

Respiratory failure is a condition characterized by inadequate oxygenation and/or ventilation. It should be anticipated in any child who shows an increased respiratory rate and then begins to show signs of fatigue, or has an altered level of consciousness, poor muscle tone, or cyanosis. Children usually progress very quickly from respiratory distress to failure; therefore, *early intervention is crucial.*

Chapter 5 focuses on specific injuries that may cause breathing problems in the child and their appropriate management.

Circulation

The circulation should be assessed as discussed in Chapter 6.

Brief Neurologic Assessment

Hypoxia may lead to changes in the child's behavior. All children with mental status changes should be placed on 100% oxygen and have early, aggressive airway manage ment.

It is critical that children with an abnormal mental status be well oxygenated.

Critical Transport Decisions

All children with an unstable airway, respiratory insufficiency, or an altered mental status must be packaged rapidly and transported to an appropriate institution.

Package and Transport Interventions

It is critical that the airway be managed as early as possible. Maintenance of adequate oxygenation and ventilation are important for a good outcome for the child.

C-spine and airway. *C-spine control should be maintained throughout any airway manipulations, particularly intubation attempts.* If the child is not able to be oxygenated and ventilated with a bag–valve–mask or if the extrication is prolonged, the child should be intubated in the field. If the patient is effectively ventilated with a bag–valve–mask, intubation should be performed en route to the hospital. Have all the necessary equipment prepared prior to the intubation attempt. Suction should be easily accessible. Do not prolong suction attempts, as this may result in bradycardia from stimulation of the vagus nerve, particularly in children less than 6 months old. Endotracheal tubes one–half size smaller and one–half size larger than are expected to be appropriate for the age and size of the child should be available. All children less than 8 years old should receive an uncuffed tube. A card with the correct sizes for the various ages should be placed in the intubation box (Table 4.1). A quick way to estimate the endotracheal tube size is to use the child's nares or the size of the smallest finger. Children with a history of previous intubations, stridor, or a history of malformations of the airway can be expected to need a smaller size endotracheal tube. Hyperventilate the child with 100% oxygen prior to intubation attempts.

All pediatric intubations should be performed by the most skilled person available. If the child is easily oxygenated and ventilated with a bag–valve–mask, it may not be necessary to intubate the child prior to arrival at the hospital. The more attempts that are performed, the more damage may be inflicted on the airway. As a rule, no more than two attempts should be made by any individual. During the intubation, the Sellick maneuver, *gentle* pressure on the cricoid cartilage, may be used to close the esophagus to minimize the child's risk of aspiration. If there is any danger of c-spine injury, careful immobilization must be maintained. Endotracheal intubation is discussed in Skill Station 2.

Pulse oximetry is useful in the assessment of the oxygenation of a child. The probe should be placed on a well–perfused area, usually a finger, toe, or ear lobe, and the monitor observed. If the monitor is receiving a pulse oximetry reading correctly, the patient's pulse will correlate with the pulse seen on the monitor. All pediatric trauma victims should have a pulse oximetry reading of 100%; less than 90% is unacceptable because this correlates with an arterial PO_2 of 56 to 60 (too low). When the child is cold or is in shock (poor perfusion), pulse oximetry may not work or give inaccurate information.

Age	Endotracheal tube Size(mm)	Suction Catheter Size(F)	Endotracheal Tube Depth
Premature	2.5	5	Infants
Newborn	3.0–3.5	6–8	< 1 yr
1–6 mo	3.5–4.0	8	7+kg=__cm depth
7–12 mo	4.0–4.5	8–10	
18 mo	4.0–4.5	8–10	
3 yr	4.5–5.0	10	
6 yr	5.0	10	> 1 yr
8 yr	5.5–6.0	10	12+1/2 age=
10 yr	5.5–6.0	10	__cm depth
12 yr	6.0–6.5	10	
15 yr	6.5–8.0	10–14	

Table 4.1. Equipment size by age group.

Breathing. All children should be maintained on 100% oxygen during transport. If the child is intubated, carefully assess endotracheal tube placement. Correct positioning is supported by symmetric rise and fall of the chest, equal breath sounds bilaterally, vapor in the tube, and acceptable pulse oximetry readings. When available, in addition to pulse oximetry, end–tidal CO2 monitoring may be used and recordings documented on the chart. If the abdomen is very distended, consider placement of an orogastric tube to allow deflation of the stomach. Chapter 5 discusses specific injuries that may be discovered.

Circulation. If time permits, IV access may be obtained on all patients with respiratory compromise. If the child has signs and symptoms of shock, fluid resuscitation should be initiated. If the patient is stable, fluid administration should be kept to a minimum so that pulmonary edema does not occur.

Medications. Occasionally, sedation may be necessary to allow for maintenance of the endotracheal tube. Only short–acting nonparalytic medications should be used, unless approved by medical control. Benzodiazepines such as midazolam produce amnesia and sedation with minimal hemodynamic depression and are frequently used to sedate an intubated patient.

Secondary Survey

During the secondary survey, note any facial injuries, abrasions, bruises, or fractures. Also record any swelling or bruises to the neck. Document any fluid that is draining from the ears or nose. As discussed in Chapter 5, carefully document any bruises or injuries to the child's chest.

Points to Remember

1. The pediatric airway is different from the adult airway.
2. Early signs and symptoms of respiratory distress should be identified rapidly and managed aggressively.
3. The most common cause of cardiopulmonary arrest is respiratory arrest.
4. The most important aspect of pediatric trauma management is maintaining an open airway.

Bibliography

1. Blackwell T: Prehospital care. *Emerg Med Clin North Am* 1993;11:1.
2. Moloney–Harmon P: Initial assessment and stabilization of the critically injured child. *Crit Care Nursing Clin North Am* 1991;3:399.
3. Mazurek A: Pediatric trauma: Overview of the problem, *Post Anesthesiol Nursing* 1991;6:331–335.
4. Todres D: Pediatric airway control and ventilation. *Ann Emerg Med* 1993;22:440.

Pediatric Chest Trauma

Robert E. Falcone, MD, FACEP
Holly Herron, MSN

Introduction

In children, as in adults, up to one quarter of trauma deaths are due to thoracic injury. Although isolated chest injuries in children are rare, they may occur as part of a multisystem injury. Two thirds of patients with potentially fatal injuries reach the emergency department alive, and less than 20% of these patients will require surgery. Expedient initial evaluation and definitive care, which often start in the field, may determine whether the child survives. Children, like adults, have identical treatment priorities and management techniques. Unlike adults, however, children have unique mechanisms of injury, anatomy, pathophysiology, and resuscitative and psychosocial concerns that must be addressed for a successful outcome.

Penetrating chest trauma is rare in children, especially in the preadolescent years. Falls and motor vehicle injuries are the most common mechanisms of injury, with sports–related injury and assault far behind. The child provides a smaller target for the focus of applied energy, so that a bumper to the thorax of a small child can injure multiple systems, whereas in an adult it may injure only the rib cage.

ANATOMY/PATHOPHYSIOLOGY

The thoracic cavity of a child, like the rest of the skeleton, is incompletely calcified and provides less of a protective cage for the internal organs. In children, multiple–system involvement is the rule rather than the exception, and serious injury without external evidence of injury is quite common. This places a great importance on the mechanism of injury as a sign of significant injury in the child. The child who has sustained a significant mechanism of injury must be assumed injured until proven otherwise.

The thorax of a child extends from the base of the neck to the umbilicus. The bony cavity is formed by 12 pairs of incompletely calcified ribs that join along the spine posteriorly and with the sternum anteriorly. There is an intercostal bundle of nerve, artery, and vein that runs along the inferior border of each rib. The thoracic cavity and its contents are lined with a thin membrane called the pleura. There is a potential space between the visceral pleura on the lungs and the parietal pleura on the chest wall. This space can become filled with air (pneumothorax) or blood (hemothorax) in injury. The adult space can hold up to 3 liters of fluid. In the child, it is proportional to size.

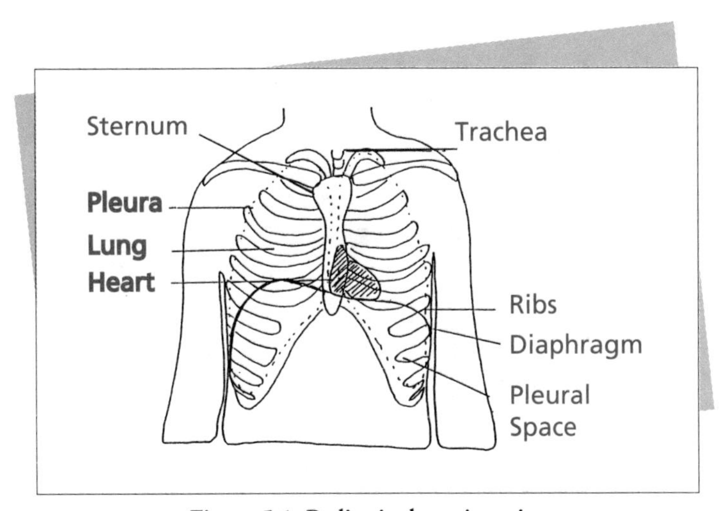

Figure 5.1. Pediatric thoracic cavity.

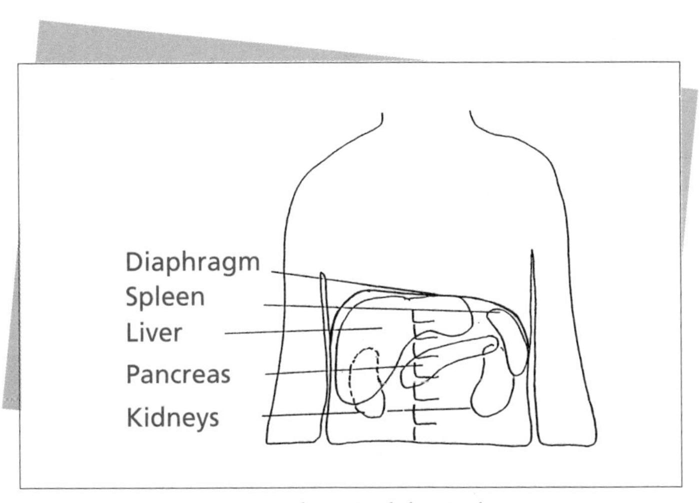

Figure 5.2. Intrathoracic abdominal contents.

Figure 5.1 is an illustration of the child's thoracic cavity and its contents. Each side of the chest contains a lung separated in the middle by the mediastinum, which contains, in order from front to back, the heart, tracheobronchial tree, superior and inferior vena cava, esophagus, aorta, and posterior spine. The chest and abdomen are separated by a muscular and ligamentous structure called the diaphragm.

The level of the diaphragm changes with inspiration and expiration, and, in general, any injury below the level of the nipples is considered not only a thoracic injury but an intraabdominal injury as well. Figure 5.2 shows the intrathoracic abdominal contents.

ASSESSMENT

The signs and symptoms of significant intrathoracic injury in a child are similar to those of an adult, but may be more subtle and should be tempered by a very high index of suspicion.

The standard approach should be followed:

1. Scene survey
2. Airway, c–spine control, and initial LOC
3. Breathing
4. Circulation
5. Brief exam of abdomen, pelvis, and extremities
6. Critical transport decisions
7. Package and transport interventions
8. Secondary survey

Scene Survey

The child with a significant mechanism of injury has a significant injury until proven otherwise. In children, this should be "The Dirty Dozen, plus one." Immediate life–threatening injuries include:

1. Airway obstruction
2. Open pneumothorax
3. Tension pneumothorax
4. Massive hemothorax
5. Flail chest
6. Cardiac tamponade
7. Thoracic aortic disruption
8. Bronchial disruption
9. Myocardial contusion
10. Diaphragmatic tear
11. Esophageal injury
12. Pulmonary contusion
13. Rib fractures

Airway and C–spine

After carefully immobilizing the child's c–spine, open the child's airway. Airway management is the first priority in the care of an injured child and is addressed in Chapter 4.

Breathing

In addition to the findings listed in Chapter 4, tachypnea, flaring, retracting, grunting, and apnea, the child with a chest injury may present with shortness of breath or pain. A small child may not be able to verbalize these complaints. If the child's airway is open and the child shows signs of respiratory distress, a rapid evaluation of the chest should be performed. This should include an evaluation of the patient's overall condition and color. Are the lips and mucous membranes pink or blue? Carefully inspect the chest for external evidence of injury. Observe the motion of the chest. Is it symmetric or not? Palpate the position of the trachea and observe the neck veins for distention. The chest should be auscultated for breath sounds. Remember that the chest wall in children is thin, so sometimes it is difficult to appreciate subtle differences in breath sounds. All children with a suspected chest injury should receive 100% oxygen and have their ventilations assisted as necessary regardless of the specific thoracic injury suspected. If available, pulse oximetry should be used to monitor the patient's oxygenation.

Chest injuries that require immediate action include open pneumothorax, tension pneumothorax, and flail chest.

Open pneumothorax. Open pneumothorax, a "sucking" chest wound, is unusual in the preadolescent child and is usually due to penetrating thoracic injury. The signs and symptoms are proportional to the chest wall defect (Figure 5.3). Normal respiration is accomplished when a negative pressure is developed in the thoracic cavity by the contracting diaphragm and expanding chest wall. Air is drawn through the upper respiratory tree and the lungs expand. A large defect in the chest wall creates a path of lesser resistance for air flow. This means that air enters the pleural space rather than the respiratory tree, making ventilation and oxygenation difficult. *Close the chest wall defect rapidly.* This is accomplished safely by using any available pad made nonocclusive by taping it on three sides. This prevents air from sucking into the thoracic cavity on inspiration, but will still allow the exit of air on expiration, helping to prevent a tension pneumothorax (Figure 5.3).

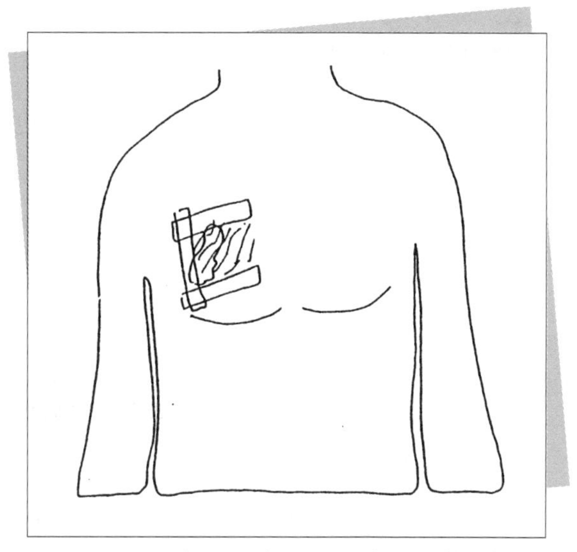

Figure 5.3. Closure of an open chest wall defect.

Tension pneumothorax. A tension pneumothorax results when a lung leak due to blunt or penetrating trauma fails to seal. A one–way valve effect may be produced, leading to air build– up in the pleural space with each breath. This can result in a shift of the mediastinum to the side opposite the tension pneumothorax with rapidly progressive dyspnea, cyanosis, and death (Figure 5.4). In young children, this may be particularly problematic, as their mobile mediastinum allows for rapid compromise of their pulmonary and cardiac function. *Early diagnosis is critical.*

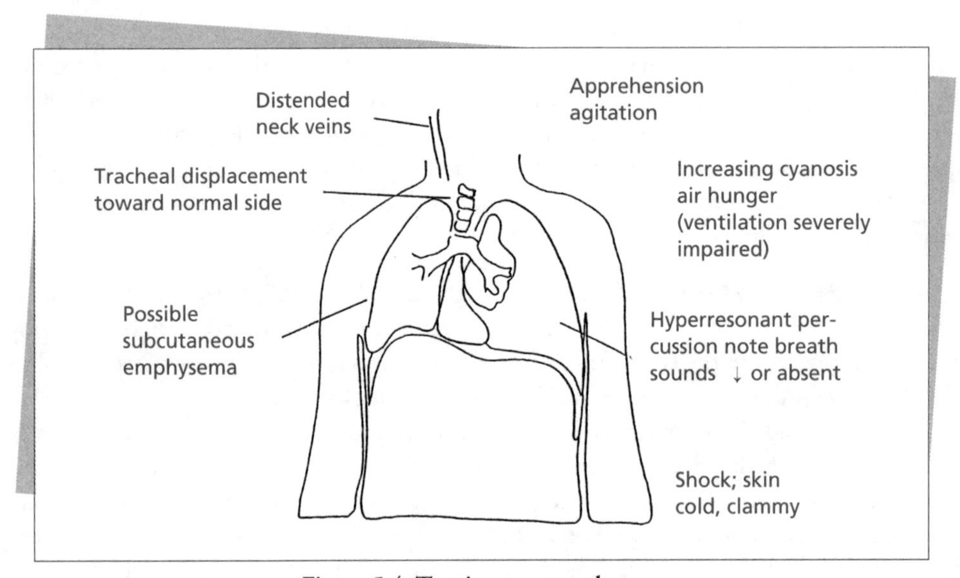

Figure 5.4. Tension pneumothorax.

Clinically, breath sounds are generally diminished on the side of the pneumothorax. However, breath sounds may be misleading in the young child, and their presence or absence should not be the sole criterion for diagnosis. Percussion may reveal hyper–resonance, although this is very unreliable in the pediatric population.

Hypotension, distended neck veins, and tracheal deviation, best appreciated by palpating the neck, occur as the process progresses and are much more reliable, but often are late findings in a child.

The chest must be decompressed by inserting an appropriately sized plastic catheter (Table 5.1) over the top of the second or third rib in the midclavicular line (Figure 5.5). If the

		Procedure	
Age (Yr)	Size (kg)	IV	Needle Decompression
<1	<10	20g	20g
1-5	10-20	18g	18g
5-12	20-40	18-16g	16g
>12	>40	14-16g	14g

Table 5.1. Age–appropriate intercaths.

catheter is left open to air, this converts a tension pneumothorax into a simple pneumothorax. Indications to perform an emergency decompression of a tension pneumothorax include loss of consciousness, severe respiratory distress, cyanosis, and traumatic cardiorespiratory arrest with evidence of chest injury. If protocols prohibit chest decompression, the patient must be immediately transported to the nearest facility. Needle decompression is a temporary option and must be replaced by chest tube placement as soon as possible.

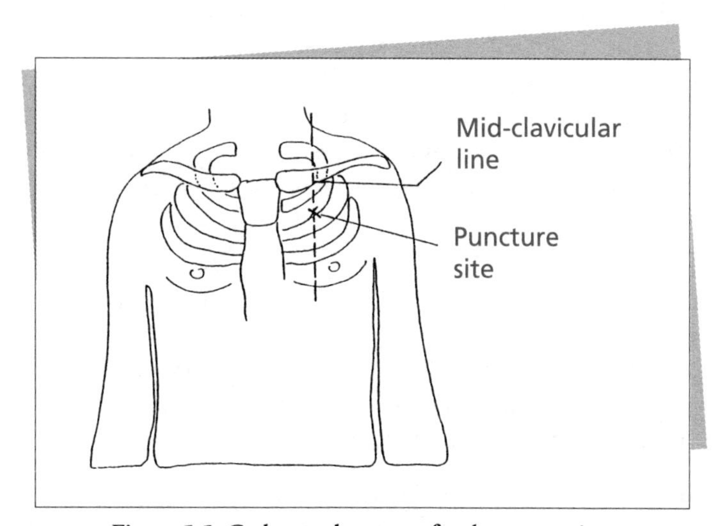

Figure 5.5. Catheter placement for decompression.

Flail chest. By definition, a flail chest occurs when three or more adjacent ribs are fractured in at least two places. This results in a segment of chest wall that is no longer mechanically contiguous with the rest of the thorax. The flail can occur laterally or anteriorly and typically

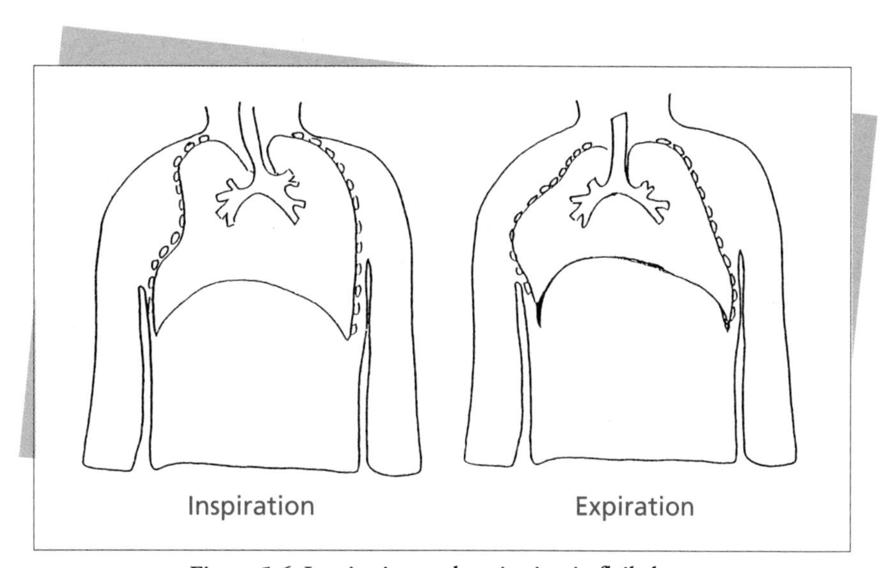

Figure 5.6. Inspiration and expiration in flail chest.

produces a paradoxical motion such that on inspiration, while the rest of the chest expands, the flail sucks in; on expiration, when the rest of the chest contracts, the flail flutters out.

In children, any number of rib fractures, not necessarily three contiguous ribs, may result in paradoxical movement of the chest (Figure 5.6).

In an adult, the paradoxical motion associated with a flail segment is not of significant consequence. Although this injury is unusual in a child, paradoxical movement associated with flail can be quite debilitating and may mandate assisted ventilation. The bigger problem, however, is that such serious injury to the chest wall is almost always associated with severe, underlying chest injury. A patient with a flail segment generally has a pulmonary contusion and is at serious risk for hemothorax, pneumothorax, and marked respiratory distress. Findings may include a visible flail segment, tenderness to palpation of the chest wall, crepitus, and respiratory distress. After the airway has been secured, assist ventilations as necessary. This frequently can be accomplished effectively in a young child with a bag–valve–mask device.

Circulation

Chest trauma may present with the combination of respiratory distress and shock. In addition, isolated chest or abdominal injury is unusual, and any findings suggestive of an abdominal injury should point to the possibility of coexistent chest injury. The two most common injuries fitting this category are hemothorax and cardiac tamponade. Prehospital management focuses on stabilization of the ABCs and transport.

Hemothorax. Blood in the pleural space is a hemothorax. The presence of large amounts of blood involving up to one half or more of one thoracic cavity is considered a massive hemothorax. Massive hemothorax, which is most often caused by penetrating rather than blunt trauma, is generally caused by disruption of a major pulmonary or systemic vessel. Blood accumulating within a pleural space compresses the lung on the affected side. If blood accumulates under pressure, the mediastinum can be shifted away from the hemothorax, resulting in a

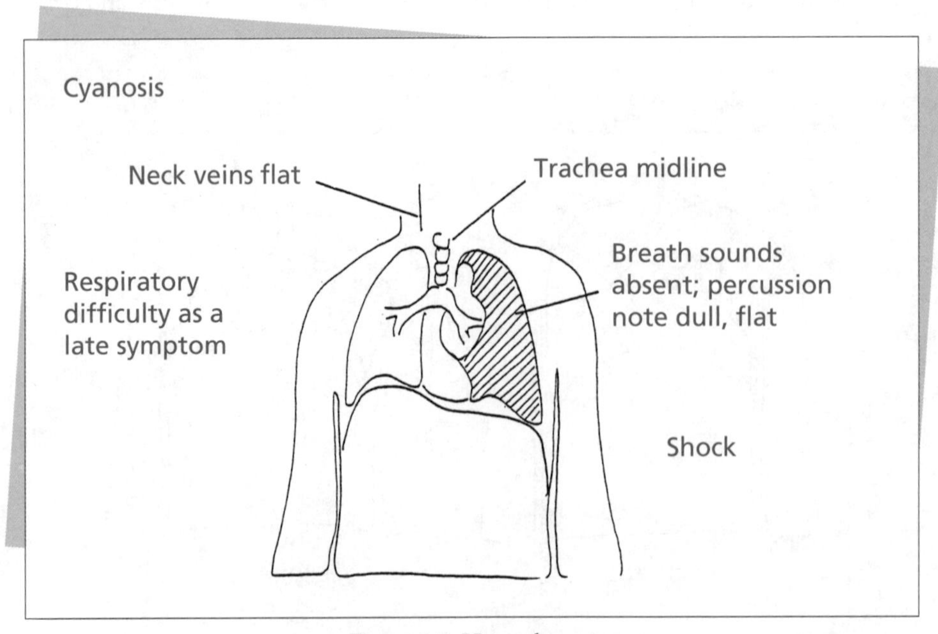

Figure 5.7. Hemothorax.

"tension" effect. Unlike tension pneumothorax, though, this cannot be relieved by needle decompression.

The signs and symptoms of massive hemothorax are primarily those of hypovolemia and respiratory compromise (Figure 5.7). Like a tension pneumothorax, the patient is generally hypotensive and in respiratory distress, and breath sounds are diminished on the affected side. However, unlike a tension pneumothorax, the chest may be dull to percussion (unreliable in children), the neck veins are generally flat, and the trachea is almost always in the midline. In the young child with a very mobile mediastinum, the neck veins can become distended and the trachea can be shifted. In this situation, it is reasonable to attempt an anterior needle decompression to rule out the presence of a tension pneumothorax. Table 5.2 provides a comparison between tension pneumothorax and massive hemothorax. After the airway and breathing have been appropriately addressed, shock must be managed, following the guidelines in Chapter 6. Monitor the child very closely.

Signs/Symptoms	Tension Pneumothorax	Hemothorax	Cardiac Tamponade
Respiratory distress	Yes	No[1]	No[1]
Shock	Yes	Yes	Yes
JVD	Yes	No	Yes
Tracheal shift	Yes	No[2]	No
Breath sounds	Decreased	Decreased	Normal
Resonance	Increased	Decreased	Normal

1: Respiratory distress may occur late in the process
2: Tracheal shift may occur late in the process

Table 5.2. Tension pneumothorax, massive hemothorax and cardiac tamponade.

Cardiac tamponade. Tamponade, which is usually due to penetrating injury, is unusual in preadolescent children. The heart is surrounded by the pericardial sac, an inelastic membrane. If the potential space between the heart and the pericardium fills with air, blood, or fluid, normal cardiac mechanics are disrupted and severe hemodynamic derangement can occur. As this space fills with fluid, the heart is compressed, limiting diastolic filling. This then limits cardiac output and may result in poor perfusion and hypotension. Signs and symptoms include the diagnostic triad of hypotension, distended neck veins, and muffled heart tones. A patient also may have a paradoxical pulse, which can be evidenced by the loss of peripheral pulse during inspiration. Cardiac tamponade is sometimes difficult to distinguish from a tension pneumothorax (Table 5.2). Rapidly stabilize the ABCs and prepare to transport the patient. *This injury is rapidly fatal and cannot be readily treated in the prehospital setting.* Rapid package and transport are crucial. Figure 5.8 summarizes the pathophysiology and physical findings of cardiac tamponade.

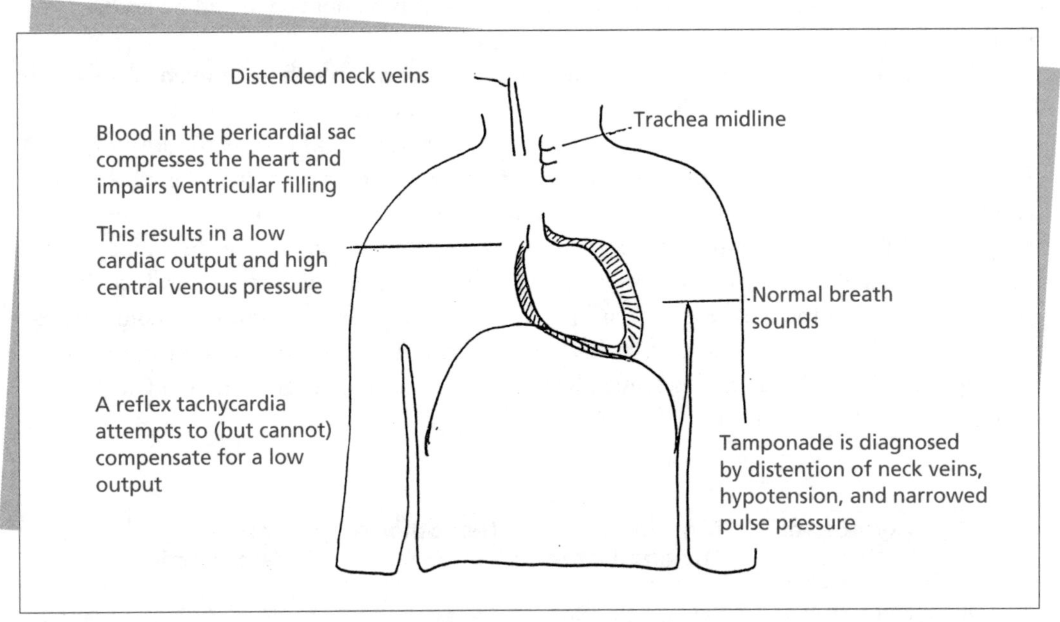

Figure 5.8. Cardiac tamponade.

Critical Transport Decisions

Any child with an unstable injury, insufficient respirations, shock, or an altered mental status should be rapidly packaged and transported. If the child has an open pneumothorax, tension pneumothorax, hemothorax, or a flail chest, extra care should be taken to expedite transport.

Package and Transport Interventions

The child should be rapidly and appropriately packaged for transport. Any child who has received a chest injury should be monitored with a cardiac monitor, for possible injury to the heart, and pulse oximetry. All children should be on 100% oxygen and maintain oxygen saturations of 95% to 100%.

Airway and c-spine. All intubations should be performed en route to the receiving facility, unless the airway cannot be stabilized with a bag–valve–mask or the child requires a prolonged extrication.

Breathing. If the patient is being ventilated, the provider may notice a decrease in lung compliance with difficulty in squeezing the bag. Children are especially prone to barotrauma, and the provider should be vigilant to the possibility of tension pneumothorax in anyone receiving assisted ventilation. Pulse oximetry will provide a continual assessment of the patient's oxygenation.

Circulation. All children with a chest injury should have continuous cardiac monitoring. Although uncommon in pediatric patients, children with a chest injury occasionally will have an associated cardiac injury and may develop arrhythmias. If time allows, IV access may be established en route to the hospital. If the child has signs or symptoms of shock, appropriate fluid resuscitation, as discussed in Chapter 6, should be instituted. The use of pneumatic anti–shock garment is not appropriate in thoracic injury and should not be used for the child with a suspected chest injury. Inflation of the abdominal compartment may further compromise the respiratory status of the child.

Secondary Survey

Complete a secondary survey if time allows. Some children with chest trauma need to have their injuries identified in the field, but the majority of their management will occur at the hospital. A comprehensive list of injuries is included below.

Traumatic aortic rupture. Traumatic aortic rupture is the most common cause of sudden death in motor vehicle accidents or falls from heights in adults. It is relatively uncommon in young children because of their elastic and mobile aortas. However, when it does occur in a child, it is almost always fatal. For survivors, salvage is possible with prompt diagnosis and surgery. Signs and physical findings in the prehospital setting are limited, but a high level of suspicion should be maintained in a child with a deceleration injury or significant thoracoabdominal injury. Upper–extremity hypertension and diminished lower–extremity pulses are rare findings. Assure a patent airway, administer 100% oxygen, and rapidly transport to the nearest appropriate facility. In addition, IV access may be obtained en route to the hospital and the EKG carefully monitored for signs of dysrhythmia.

Tracheal or bronchial tree injury. This injury may result from either blunt or penetrating trauma and is relatively rare, even more so in young children than in adults. Definitive management is difficult in the prehospital setting, and a high index of suspicion will allow for early diagnosis and treatment once the appropriate facility is reached. Disruption of the trachea or bronchus often results in subcutaneous emphysema and tension pneumothorax. Treatment in the field should be aimed at managing these entities. Again, the focus should be on the rapid package and transport of the patient after stabilization of the airway and administration of 100% oxygen. The patient should be monitored carefully for the development of a tension pneumothorax and arrhythmias.

Myocardial contusion. This is an unusual and much overdiagnosed entity in adults and is very rare in children, but it is a consideration in any patient suffering blunt chest injury. Blunt injury to the central chest can result in a bruise or contusion to the heart. Abnormalities can range from mild tachycardia to cardiovascular collapse. Symptoms may be absent or include chest pain and shortness of breath. Findings may include external evidence of injury, tachycardia, or abnormalities on EKG. Stabilize the patient's ABCs and remember to monitor for development of arrhythmias. Be prepared to treat dysrhythmias as they occur per ACLS protocols.

Diaphragmatic injury. Traumatic diaphragmatic injury can occur in thoracoabdominal penetrating injury or from any severe blunt injury to the thorax or abdomen that results in a sudden increase in intra–abdominal pressure. This may include seatbelt injuries, kicks to the abdomen, falls, or crush injuries. A blunt or penetrating force leads to a tear in the diaphragm. Intra–abdominal pressure, which is generally positive, overcomes intrapleural pressure, which is generally negative, forcing intra–abdominal contents into the chest.

This can compromise blood supply to the intra–abdominal contents and diminish ventilatory capacity of the affected lung. Ruptures tend to occur much more often in the left side than the right side and are difficult to diagnose in the prehospital setting. Symptoms may include chest or abdominal pain and shortness of breath. Findings may include external evidence of thoracoabdominal penetrating or blunt injury, abnormalities in chest wall excursion or ventilatory rate, diminished breath sounds in the chest, or bowel sounds heard in the chest. The abdomen on occasion appears scaphoid if a large quantity of the abdominal content has entered the chest. After stabilization of the ABCs, rapidly package and transport the patient. Placement of a nasogastric tube en route to the receiving facility may be considered if time allows.

Esophageal injury. Esophageal injury is rare and almost always due to penetrating injury. Its diagnosis in the prehospital setting is not generally possible, and management should be limited to the associated trauma.

Pulmonary contusion. Pulmonary contusion is the most common form of injury following blunt trauma and, in the child, may occur with no external evidence of injury. It should be based on a high index of suspicion and treated in the prehospital setting with supportive care. Special attention should be given to maintaining oxygen saturations above 95%.

Rib fractures. Rib fractures in the child, even when isolated, carry a very high mortality rate and should be treated as a sign of serious injury. Rib fractures are usually associated with a high degree of force generated to cause such an injury. This extreme force causes underlying lung damage. Fractures of the first and second ribs are often associated with vascular injury; fractures of the ninth through twelfth ribs are often associated with intra–abdominal injury. The management should be to provide supportive care and to realize that these injuries are a strong indicator of severe trauma in the child.

Other injuries. Other thoracic injuries in the child may include impalement injuries, traumatic asphyxia, thoracic spine injury, sternal fracture, and simple pneumothorax.

Impalement injuries should be treated as impalement injuries anywhere,i.e., the impaled object should be left in place and protected. Associated abnormalities should be dealt with as appropriate. It is important to remember that, depending on the object and the location, there is a potential for development of any of the injuries previously mentioned.

Traumatic asphyxia is a physical finding and a misnomer because the condition is not caused by asphyxia. The syndrome results from a severe compression injury to the chest such as compression under a heavy object. The sudden pressure on the heart and mediastinum transmits this force to the capillaries of the head and neck and results in cyanosis above the level of the compression with swelling of the head and neck, capillary hemorrhage, and discoloration. Traumatic asphyxia indicates that the patient has suffered severe blunt injury and should be an indication that significant underlying trauma may be present.

Thoracic spine and sternal fractures are also indications that the patient has suffered severe injury and should be treated as such. In addition, the potential for thoracic spine injury should be dealt with by appropriate spinal immobilization. Sternal fractures are often associated with myocardial contusions, so monitor the patient en route to the hospital for dysrhythmias.

Simple pneumothorax, which is generally well tolerated by adults, may not be so easily tolerated by children. A simple pneumothorax should be suspected if breath sounds are diminished and the child is in respiratory distress. Increased resonance is an unreliable indicator in pediatric patients. Patients with a simple pneumothorax should be prepared for emergency needle decompression during transport if a tension pneumothorax develops.

Points to Remember

1. Isolated chest injuries are uncommon in children, they are usually associated with multisystem injury.
2. A child may have severe underlying injury with relatively little external evidence of trauma.
3. The basics of management remain the same as in the adult and include ensuring a patent airway while protecting the c–spine, administration of high concentrations of oxygen, needle decompression if needed, appropriate backboard stabilization, IV access, EKG monitoring, rapid transport to the appropriate facility, and notification of medical control.

Suggested Reading

1. Baffes TG: Thoracic trauma, in Raffensperger JG (ed): *Swenson's Pediatric Surgery.* New York, Appleton–Century–Crofts, 1980, p 226–227.
2. Garcia VF, Gotschall CS, et al: Rib fractures in children: A marker of severe trauma. *J Trauma* 1990;30:695.
3. Harris GJ, Soper RT: Pediatric first rib fractures. *J Trauma* 1990;30:343.
4. Kilman JW, Charnock E: Thoracic trauma in infancy and childhood. *J Trauma* 1969;9:863–873.
5. Mattox KL, Bickell W, Pepe PE, et al: Prospective MAST study in 911 patients. *J Trauma* 1989;29:1104.
6. O'Neill JA: Infants and children as accident victims, in Welch JA, Randolph JG, Ravitch MM, et al (eds): *Pediatric Surgery.* Chicago, Year Book Medical Publishers, 1986, p 133–135.
7. Polley TZ, Coran AC: Special problems in management of pediatric trauma. *Crit Care Clin* 1986;2:775.
8. Sinclair MC, Moore TC: Major surgery for abdominal and thoracic trauma in childhood and adolescence. *J Pediat Surg* 1974;9:155–162.
9. Smyth BT: Chest trauma in children. *J Pediat Surg* 1979;14:41–47.
10. Yurt RW: Triage, initial assessment, and early treatment of the pediatric trauma patient. *Pediat Emerg Med* 1992;39:1083–1091.
11. Zorludemir U, Ergoren Y, Selcuk Y, et al: Mortality due to trauma in childhood. *J Trauma* 1988;28:669–671.

Pediatric Shock and Fluid Resuscitation

Linda Manley, RN
Kathy J. Haley, RN

Introduction

After carefully attending to the child's airway and ventilation, the next priority becomes assessment of circulation. Hypovolemia, an acute loss of blood volume, is the most common cause of shock in children and a leading cause of death. Shock results from inadequate tissue perfusion and oxygen delivery. Signs of shock in children are subtle and must be recognized and treated aggressively for a good patient outcome. This chapter reviews the signs and symptoms of hypovolemic shock in children and identifies prehospital management strategies.

ANATOMY/PATHOPHYSIOLOGY

Children are not small adults. This becomes most evident when assessing them for acute loss of blood. Children are very adept at compensating — possibly too adept. Although they may initially appear "stable," they may "crash" very quickly due to cardiovascular collapse.

Even before the assessment begins, it is important to recognize normal pediatric vital signs and be able to estimate a child's circulating blood volume (CBV). This knowledge can greatly simplify resuscitation. The CBV of a child is based on body weight and averages about 80 mL/kg. Thus, a 2–year–old child weighing 12 kg has a CBV of 960 mL, or roughly 1 liter of fluid. Loss of only a few hundred milliliters can be life–threatening. It is important to consider not only the visible external blood loss, from lacerations, abrasions, and the like, but also the potential internal losses from major organ injuries.

In general, children can tolerate a loss of 10% to 15% of their CBV with minimal signs and symptoms. A loss of more than 15% of CBV, however, activates the "flight or fight" response. Epinephrine, a potent catecholamine, is secreted and causes intense vasoconstriction and tachycardia, both of which help maintain the systolic blood pressure.[1] With a significant blood loss, however, the child's cardiac output diminishes, and eventually cardiovascular collapse will occur if not corrected rapidly.

ASSESSMENT

As mentioned, in Chapter 2, the mechanism of injury is important when determining the potential injuries the patient may have sustained.

In general, all patients should be evaluated in the following manner:

1. Scene survey
2. Airway, c–spine control, and initial LOC
3. Breathing
4. Circulation
5. Brief exam of abdomen, pelvis, and extremities
6. Critical transport decisions
7. Package and transport interventions
8. Secondary survey

Scene Survey

Refer to previous chapters.

Airway and C–spine

As stressed in Chapter 4, this should be of primary concern. Sometimes spinal cord injuries may result in a type of shock called neurogenic (spinal) shock, which is discussed in Chapter 7. Make sure that c–spine control is maintained throughout the assessment and management of the child.

Breathing

All children in shock should receive 100% oxygen and have their respiratory status carefully monitored. Children in shock may also exhibit tachypnea as the body tries to maximize oxygen intake. *The importance of administering 100% oxygen cannot be overemphasized.* As mentioned, shock is defined simply as inadequate tissue oxygenation; thus, the mainstay of therapy is to improve oxygenation. A child will not be harmed by receiving too much oxygen in the field.

Circulation

Early signs and symptoms of hypovolemic shock in children are subtle. Tachycardia is due to the effect of epinephrine (remember age–dependent heart rates). Altered "skin vital signs" are mottled, pale skin with slow capillary refill. (Normal capillary refill is less than 2 seconds after 5 seconds of pressure to the skin.) The strength of the pulses diminishes as the symptoms of shock progress. The child first loses peripheral pulses (radial, dorsalis pedis, and posterior tibial) and keeps central pulses (femoral, carotid, and brachial). In late shock, the child may even lose central pulses. A blood pressure reading on a child can be very difficult to obtain in the field and should be obtained en route to the hospital. In general, *shock is best recognized in a child as tachycardia and poor perfusion.*

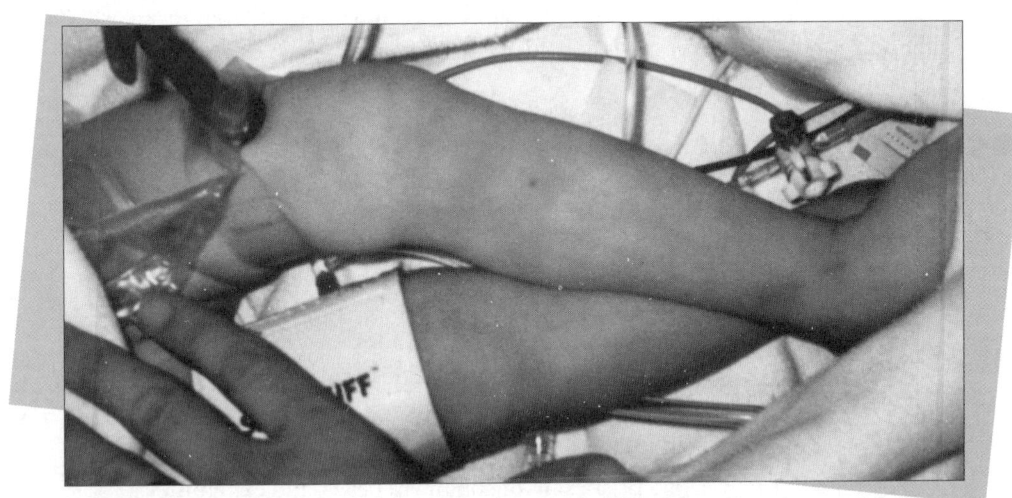

Figure 6.1. A femoral intraosseous line placed in a child with extreme poor perfusion.

Control bleeding. As the circulatory assessment is being performed, any evidence of external bleeding should be noted and carefully controlled. It is surprising how much blood loss can occur from a simple scalp laceration, especially in a child. Direct manual pressure to the laceration is often effective in minimizing blood loss. Remember also to consider internal losses, such as bleeding into a fracture site or the abdominal cavity.

Brief Neurologic Assessment

Often children with signs and symptoms of shock may appear agitated and restless due to poor circulation to their brain. Conduct a brief neurologic assessment, and if the child has an altered mental status, prepare for a rapid transport. *Remember that hypoxia can also cause mental status changes.* Maintain a patent airway and administer 100% oxygen.

Critical Transport Decisions

Children presenting with signs and symptoms of hypovolemic shock need to be transported rapidly, ideally to a pediatric trauma center. During the transport, the ABCs must be continually assessed and reassessed.

Package and Transport Interventions

Airway and c–spine. Provide care as discussed in Chapter 4.

Breathing. Maintain the child on high concentrations of oxygen. Continually reassess the patient for signs of respiratory failure that may accompany shock. If respiratory failure develops, manage as discussed in Chapter 4.

Circulation. If you have time and can obtain a blood pressure, do so en route to the hospital. Compare it with the normal range of blood pressures for age (at a minimum, 70 + 2 x age for systolic blood pressure). *It is important to remember that hypotension is a late sign of shock in children.* It takes a loss of 30% to 35% of the CBV before hypotension occurs. *Hypotension is an ominous finding.*

Another method to control blood loss is the pneumatic antishock garment, also known as military antishock trousers (MAST). MAST are very controversial and their use in pediatrics has not been well researched. In general, the MAST work well to splint lower–extremity fractures and stabilize pelvic fractures. The abdominal compartment can interfere with ventilation by limiting diaphragmatic excursion (remember, the diaphragm is the primary muscle of respiration in children) and precipitating vomiting and possibly aspiration. *Children who have a marginal respiratory effort may progress to respiratory failure with inflation of the abdominal compartment.*

MAST are available in the following sizes: toddler, for ages less than 6 years; pediatric, ages 6 to 10 years; and adult, ages 10 years and up.

Establish IV access en route to the receiving facility. Establishing access can be difficult and time–consuming in a healthy child, let alone one who is hypovolemic. If IV access is indicated, over–the–needle catheters can be started in the hand, forearm, or antecubital fossa. Another site that usually is easily accessible is the saphenous vein. Use the largest catheter diameter with the shortest length. The prehospital care provider often will be successful using a catheter one size larger than originally anticipated.

The truly hypovolemic child will most likely present with mottled, cold extremities and unstable vital signs. In this case, vascular access may be possible only by an alternate route, intraosseous infusion. Intraosseous infusion is the infusion of fluids, blood, and/or drugs directly into the bone marrow cavity. In the field and emergency department settings, it is becoming an increasingly popular route for venous access if the child is *unstable.* Some authors[3] advocate that an intraosseous infusion should be started after two *quick* peripheral attempts in a patient who is in cardiopulmonary arrest, unconscious, or in severe shock.

It is important to understand the basic principles of intraosseous infusion. Fluids enter directly into the bone marrow cavity and are absorbed into the central circulation by a network of venous sinusoids. In children less than 4 years old, the bone marrow cavity is responsible for the production of red blood cells. After this age, some fat cells occupy the marrow cavity of the long bones, gradually filling them with yellow "fatty" marrow. Fortunately, serious complications are rare with this procedure if done correctly.

The sites of choice for an intraosseous infusion are the long bones of the lower extremity. The most frequent site for insertion is the anterior proximal medial aspect of the tibia, 1 to 3 cm below the tibial tuberosity, as there are no vital structures that could be injured (Figure 6.2). Absolute contraindications are a fracture of the bone or unsuccessful prior attempt. An alternative site is the distal third of the anterior femur, although there is a greater muscle mass at this site.

Once the IV or intraosseous line is established, it should be taped securely and immobilized properly so that it does not become dislodged. All medications, fluids, and even blood can be administered safely through the intraosseous route. This technique will be further addressed in Skill Station 3.

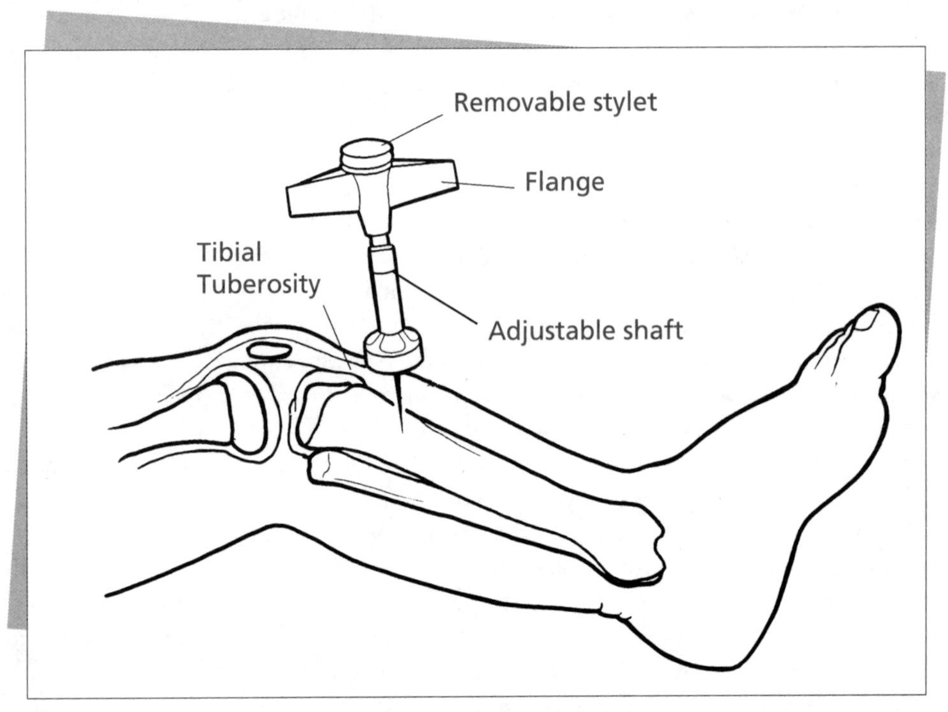

Figure 6.2. Intraosseous infusion.

Initiate fluid resuscitation. Rapid administration of fluids is essential in the treatment of hypovolemic shock. IV or intraosseous access should be attempted en route to the hospital. It is important to begin aggressive fluid resuscitation en route to the hospital. If the child requires a prolonged extrication, fluid resuscitation may be initiated on the scene. The fluid of choice is Ringer's lactate or normal saline. Fluids are administered to children by a fluid bolus, a predetermined amount based on the child's weight.

A fluid bolus is given as a rapid way to correct hypovolemia. The child's response to the bolus can be an early, reliable indicator of continued blood loss. For example, most children who receive a fluid bolus will show marked improvement. If that does not happen, consider ongoing blood loss. If there is evidence of shock (tachycardia and delayed capillary refill), 20 mL/kg can be administered safely. If the child continues to exhibit signs of shock and/or is hypotensive, administer an additional 20 mL/kg. The bolus may be repeated again if indicated by medical control. On arrival at the hospital, report the total volume of fluids that have been administered. Since the condition of head-injured children can be worsened by inadequate profusion, it is critical to administer fluids to a child with head injury *and shock*.

Thermal regulation. Children are prone to hypothermia because of their greater body surface area and lack of subcutaneous tissue. Administer warm fluids whenever possible, and keep the child wrapped between assessments and during transport.

Secondary Survey

Complete a secondary survey, looking carefully for sources of blood loss. An abdominal or pelvic injury may result in shock in a pediatric patient. These injuries cannot be corrected in the field and require close management at a pediatric center.

Points to Remember

1. Shock is defined as inadequate tissue oxygenation. Hypovolemic shock is the most common type of shock in children.
2. Subtle, early signs of hypovolemic shock include tachycardia, weakness of the peripheral pulses, poor peripheral perfusion (capillary refill of more than 2 seconds, pallor, or mottled skin), tachypnea, and agitation or restlessness. Hypotension is a late and ominous sign of shock.
3. External blood loss should be controlled with direct pressure. The MAST should be used cautiously.
4. IV or intraosseous access can be life–saving. Intraosseous infusion can be used to administer fluids, blood, and/or drugs directly into the bone marrow cavity and is most often done on the young child.
5. Once vascular access has been established, an isotonic solution should be administered by a fluid bolus (20 mL/kg), and the child should be reevaluated carefully. If there is no improvement, a second bolus (same amount) should be administered. The receiving hospital should be notified of the child's response.
6. It is important to reassess ABCs frequently and ensure that the child does not become hypothermic.
7. Rapid transport to a pediatric trauma center is indicated for children with signs and symptoms of hypovolemic shock, especially those who do not respond to one fluid bolus.

Bibliography

1. Committee on Trauma: *Advanced Trauma Life Support.* Chicago, American College of Surgeons, 1988.
2. Strange G: Pediatric resuscitation, in Callaham ML (ed): *Current Practice of Emergency Medicine.* Philadelphia, BC Decker, 1991, p1206–1214.
3. Manley L, Haley KJ, Dick MR: Intraosseous infusion: Rapid vascular access for critically ill or injured infants and children. *J Emerg Nursing* 1988; 14:63-69.
4. Colombani P, Haller JA: The pediatric trauma patient, in Callaham ML (ed): *Current Practice of Emergency Medicine.* Philadelphia, BC Decker, 1991, p1215–1217.

Pediatric Spinal Trauma

David Keseg, MD, FACEP

Introduction

Spinal cord trauma is extremely uncommon in preadolescent children. Only 1% to 3.3% of all spinal injuries occur in patients less than 16 years old.[1] However rare it may be, failure to recognize the injury may result in devastating consequences for the child and the family.

Most acute spinal injuries occur during a motor vehicle accident or sporting incident. As the child approaches adolescence, more motorcycle and automobile accidents occur, leading to a higher incidence of spinal trauma with a pattern similar to that in adults. *Of utmost importance to the prehospital provider is avoidance of any injury to the child's spinal cord from the time of the accident until treatment at the hospital is complete.*

ANATOMY/PHYSIOLOGY

The spine of a child is not simply a small adult spine. The anatomy, physiology, and response to trauma are very different. The child's head is relatively large compared to the rest of the body. This may cause a force directed at the head to be transmitted through the neck, resulting in a c–spine injury. The neck is short compared to that of an adult, which limits its mobility when undergoing stress from trauma. Finally, the ligaments that support the cervical spine in a child are relatively loose and may permit too much movement of the neck when the child is "thrown around," resulting in devastating injuries. Because of these anatomic factors, most c–spine fractures in children will involve the upper portion of the cervical spine.

Although most spinal injuries that occur in the first decade of life involve the cervical region, children also may sustain thoracic and lumbar spinal injuries. These injuries usually will occur at the level of T_{11}–L_2 because this is where the relatively rigid thoracic elements adjoin the more mobile lumbar segments. In an automobile accident involving a frontal impact, a child restrained in a standard rear–seat lapbelt may sustain a mid–lumbar spinal fracture (Figure 7.1). External belt–shaped abrasions to the child's lower abdomen are important clues to a possible lumbar spine injury. Recent reports also have indicated that visceral injury may accompany this type of spinal trauma.

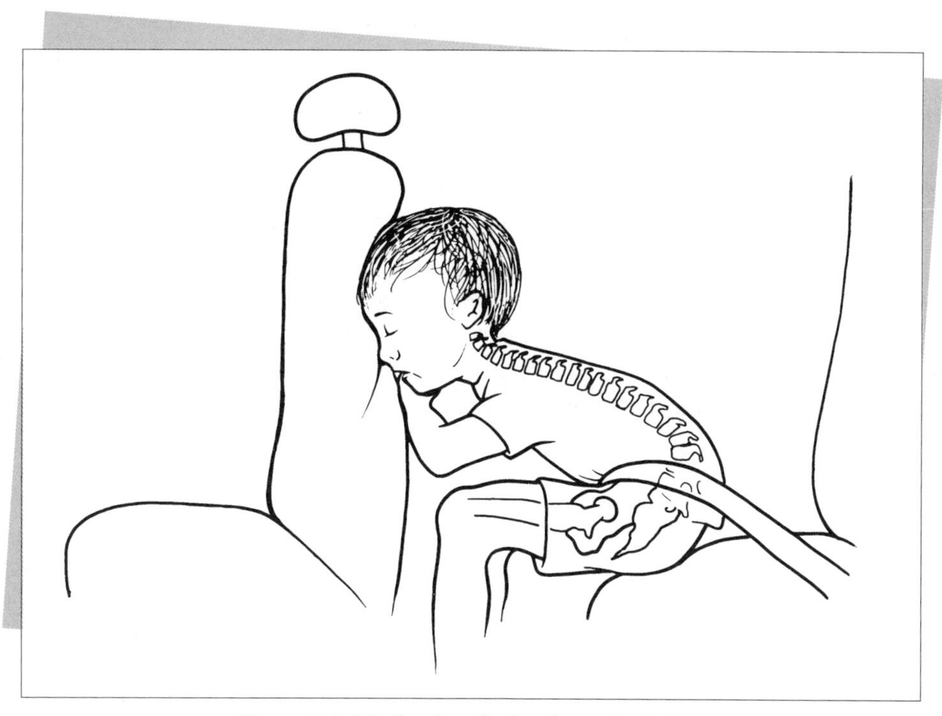

Figure 7.1. Mechanism for lumbar spine injury.

ASSESSMENT

All children should be stabilized in the same manner:

1. Scene survey
2. Airway, c–spine control, and initial LOC
3. Breathing
4. Circulation
5. Brief exam of abdomen, pelvis, and extremities
6. Critical transport decisions
7. Package and transport interventions
8. Secondary survey

Scene Survey

Any child who suffers a traumatic injury should be considered to have a spinal injury until proven otherwise. *All children should have the spine protected regardless of mechanism of injury.* Situations in which neck injuries are more likely to occur include motor vehicle–pedestrian accidents, falls from great heights, bicycle accidents, and sports injuries.

Children with head trauma or an altered mental status (drugs or alcohol) are particularly likely to have a coexistent c–spine injury; take extra care to protect their spines.

Airway and C-spine

While maintaining c–spine control, assess the airway. The initial immobilization should be with the rescuer's hands. Speak calmly to the child as the neck is firmly held in the neutral position. If the child has sustained a severe neck injury, the provider may be able to palpate a step–off on the back of the neck during the examination.

Assess the child's airway. If the airway is unstable and requires an immediate intervention, proceed as directed in Chapter 4, but remember to *maintain c–spine control.*

Breathing

Carefully assess the child's breathing. Remember, a child with an upper c–spine injury will lose the ability to breathe (apnea). This usually occurs if the injury is above the level of C5, which results in the loss of function of the phrenic and intercostal nerves. A child who is not breathing must be rapidly assisted with bag–valve–mask ventilations as discussed in Chapter 4. All patients with a suspected spinal injury should receive 100% oxygen (to keep the spinal cord well oxygenated). Continue to maintain c–spine control.

Circulation

As discussed in Chapter 6, it is important to assess the child's pulse rate, perfusion, and blood pressure (if time is available) to determine if the patient is showing signs of shock. The most common cause of shock in the pediatric trauma patient is hypovolemia. *All shock recognized in the field should be treated as hypovolemic shock.* Occasionally, a child with an upper c–spine injury will develop spinal shock, a special type of shock in which the patient is hypotensive, normothermic, and has a low heart rate. Because spinal shock is a diagnosis of exclusion, these patients should be treated as if they are hypovolemic until a definitive diagnosis can be made at the hospital.

Brief neurologic assessment. The likelihood of a c–spine injury increases with a head injury. The unconscious trauma victim carries a 15% to 20% risk of spinal column damage. Any child with an altered mental status should have the c–spine carefully protected until a definitive evaluation can be done at the hospital. Any awake and alert child who complains of neck pain must have c–spine control maintained.

Critical Transport Decisions

Any child with an *unstable airway, obvious respiratory insufficiency, shock, or an altered mental status* requires rapid package and transport to the nearest pediatric facility.

Package and Transport Interventions

Airway and c–spine. Recent studies have indicated that oral endotracheal intubations can be performed safely even in patients with spinal injuries as long as manual in–line stabilization is maintained throughout the procedure. As indicated in Chapter 4, if a child can be effectively oxygenated and ventilated using a bag–valve–mask, intubation may be delayed until arrival at the hospital. Always supply the patient with 100% oxygen. Remember that surgical cricothyroidotomy is not indicated in children less than 12 years old.

The spine should be immobilized for transport. A cervical collar may be used as long as the *appropriate* size is available. Place it carefully on the child. Because collars alone do not provide effective immobilization of a child's neck,[2] other supplemental devices must be used. If an appropriate–size collar is not available (especially in children less than 1 year old) towels may be used to immobilize the child in the neutral position. The child must be secured to a rigid spine board. The torso and lower body should be secured while manual c–spine control of the child in the collar continues. Once the body has been secured, the head may be immobilized using a head immobilizer, towel rolls, or whatever is available. As mentioned earlier, a child has a larger

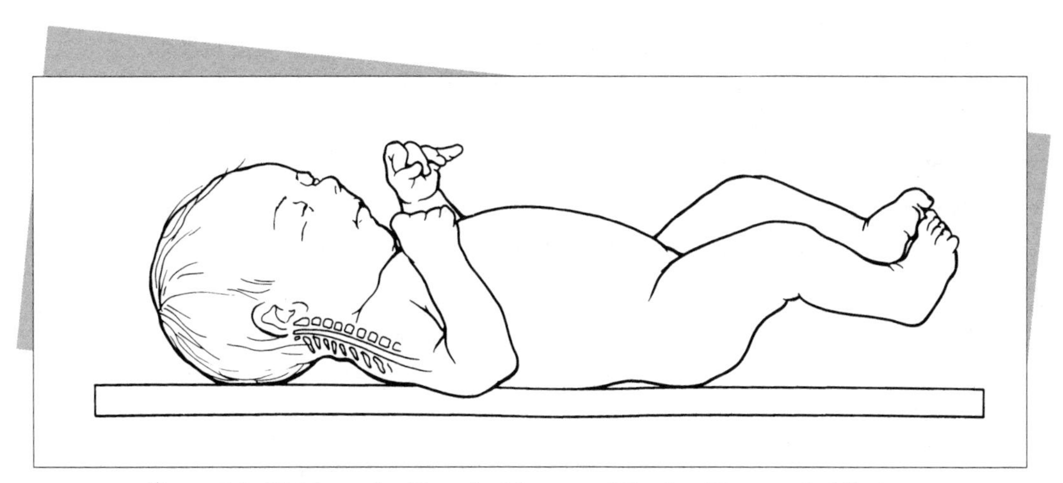

Figure 7.2. Child on a backboard without modification. Note cervical flexion.

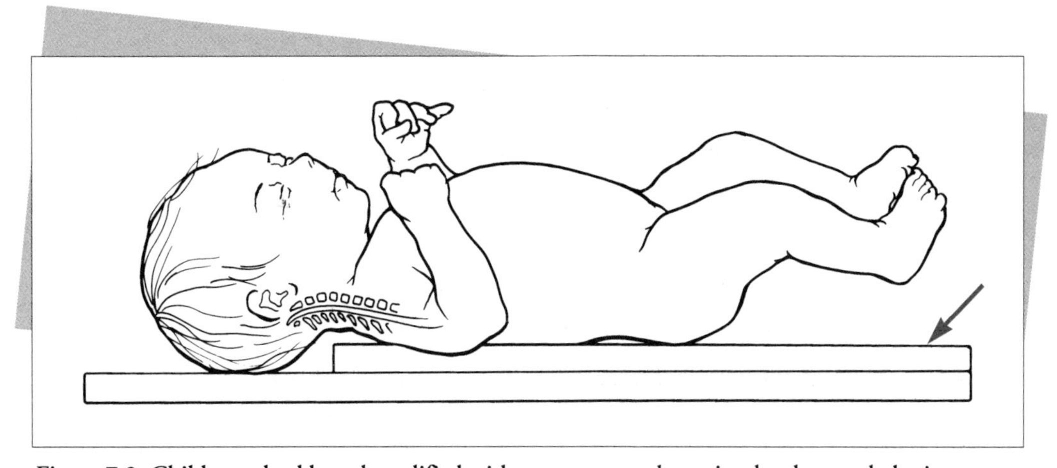

Figure 7.3. Child on a backboard modified with a mattress pad to raise the chest and obtain "neutral" positioning.

head than an adult compared to the rest of the body (Figure 7.2). To correct for this difference when using a rigid board, padding must be placed under the child's shoulders to place the neck in the "neutral" position (Figure 7.2). This should be placed on the board prior to placing it under the child.

Children in car seats must be managed cautiously. A primary assessment should be performed with the child in the seat.

If there is any compromise in the level of consciousness or ABCs, the child should be extricated. One person should stabilize the neck from above, while the other helps move the child from below. Maintain c–spine control during the time the child is being removed from the seat. Immobilize with a cervical collar, cervical immobilization device (i.e., towel rolls), and secure to a rigid spine board using padding to offset any possible c–spine flexion. *Always be sure the child's neck is in the neutral position, regardless of how secured.*

If there is no compromise to the ABCs or level of consciousness and the child is going to be transported for evaluation, he may be left in the seat. Apply a cervical collar and towel rolls, and tape the child's head securely to the seat. When a child is completely packaged, it is easy to think of the child as being "fine." However, a significant number of children in car seats may sustain serious injury. Perform a complete secondary examination with particular attention to the ABCs.

If the car seat is attached to the car, the child must be removed. The child then can be placed on a backboard and the c–spine immobilized after the assessment has been performed.

Log roll a pediatric patient as you would an adult (see Skill Station 1). During the log roll, carefully evaluate the child's back, as you would an adult's.

Breathing. A significant number of children with spinal injuries will have associated head injuries. If the child's ventilations are being assisted, hyperventilate to lower the pressure in the head.

Circulation. If the child shows signs of shock, follow the recommendations in Chapter 6. Military antishock trousers may be placed on the patient after a careful survey has been performed. In children, only the leg compartments should be inflated. If possible, start two IV lines en route to the facility. An intraosseous infusion may be considered for children in full arrest or those who have no IV access after two attempts or 90 seconds. For the pediatric patient in shock, fluid resuscitation should be initiated en route to the hospital. If the child is in shock, blood flow will be diverted from the spinal cord, which could cause further damage to an existing injury.

Secondary Survey

The secondary survey should be performed en route for patients having a compromise in the ABCs. Children being transported in car seats must have a thorough secondary examination prior to transport.

Abdominal examination. A complete examination of the abdomen also may reveal an abrasion of the lower abdomen. This should not only raise the suspicion of a visceral injury, but also suggest possible lumbar spinal trauma (Figure 7.4).

Neurologic examination. A complete neurologic assessment should be conducted as part of the secondary survey. This examination should include muscle tone and function, and sensory status. Carefully note the positioning of both the upper and lower extremities. If the patient is awake and alert, ask him to move the extremities; note the level of function so that it can be followed for improvement or deterioration.

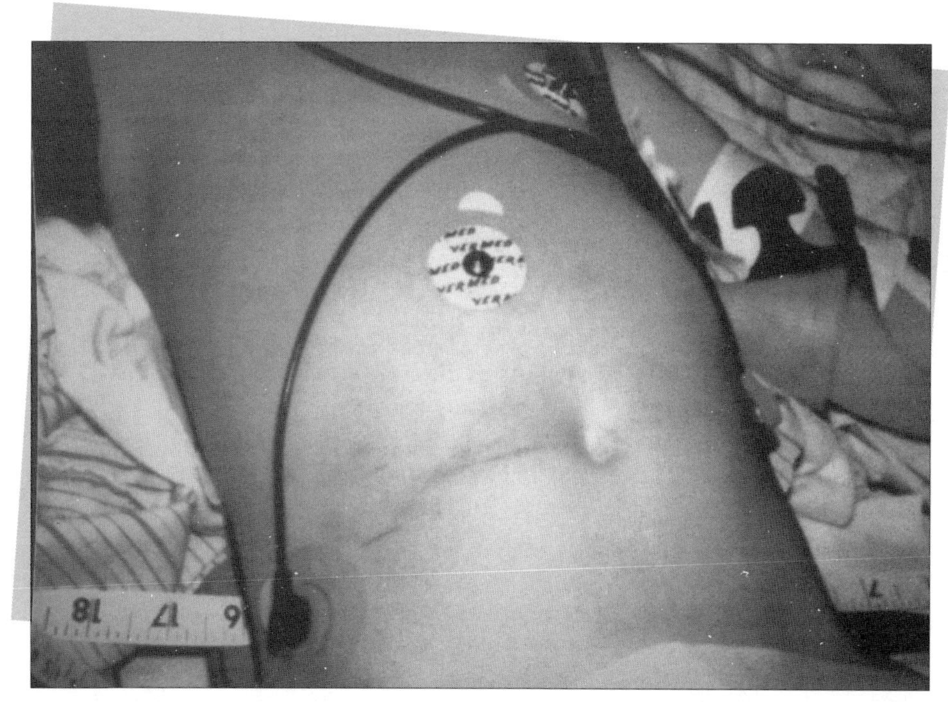

Figure 7.4. A seat belt abrasion of the abdomen suggests the possibility of lumbar spinal trauma.

A loss of function in the lower extremities with preservation of the upper extremities should suggest the presence of an injury at the thoracic or lumbar level.

Children with a complete spinal cord lesion (i.e., no sensory or motor function below the level of the injury) have a very poor prognosis for recovery of function. However, children with incomplete lesions (i.e., preservation of some function) may have complete recovery. Therefore, careful examination of the sense of position, deep pain, light touch, pinprick, and hot/cold are necessary if time allows. Reflexes will be preserved above and absent below the level of the injury.

Pharmacologic therapy. Recent studies have indicated that the administration of high–dose steroids may improve outcome in patients with a spinal cord injury if therapy is initiated early. It is crucial that spinal injuries be identified quickly and that the patient is transported to an appropriate facility.

Points to Remember

1. All children involved in a traumatic event should have their spines protected.
2. Maintain c–spine control while performing any interventions.

3. Children with spinal injuries should have their ABCs assessed rapidly, be properly packaged, and be transported to an appropriate facility.
4. Children with seat belt abrasions to their lower abdomen may have an abdominal injury and possible lumbar spinal trauma.

Bibliography

1. Fesmire F, Luten R: The pediatric cervical spine: Developmental anatomy and clinical aspects. *J Emerg Med* 1989;7:133.
2. Bohn D, Armstrong D, Becker L, et al: Cervical spine injuries in children. *J Trauma* 1990;30:463.
3. Herzenberger J, Hensiger R, Dedrick D, et al: Emergency transport and positioning of young children who have an injury of the cervical spine. *J Bone Joint Surg* 1989;71A:15– 22.
4. Stauffer S, Mazur J: Cervical spine injuries in children. *Pediatr Ann* 1982;11:6.

Pediatric Head Trauma

Laurie Lint, RN, CEN, EMT–P
Lori Dandrea, MD
Jeff Kempf, DO

Introduction

Head trauma is seen frequently in most pediatric centers, and approximately 250,000 children each year suffer some type of head injury. Although most head trauma is minor, 80% to 90% of pediatric trauma deaths are due to head trauma.

Because of the variance in growth and developmental stages that children go through, the mechanism of injury also varies with each age group. Children less than 5 years old are usually injured in the home as the result of a fall. Bicycle accidents are the most significant mechanism of head trauma in 5– to 15–year–old children. Throughout the pediatric population, just as in adults, motor vehicle accidents are the leading cause of head trauma.

ANATOMY/PHYSIOLOGY

It is important to have a basic knowledge of the anatomy of the skull and its contents to understand the various types of head injuries (Figure 8.1).

The scalp in children is highly vascularized, as it is in adults, and is a common site for lacerations. A young child may lose a significant amount of blood from even a simple laceration. Occasionally, this may even result in shock. Fortunately, direct pressure is usually adequate to

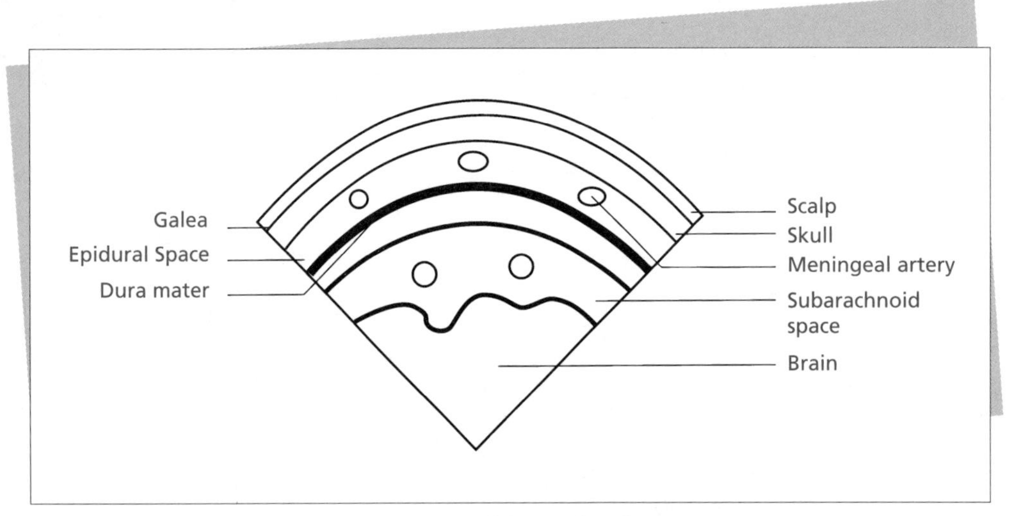

Figure 8.1. Anatomy of the skull and its contents.

control the bleeding. The lower layer of the scalp, the galea, is also a potential site for bleeding. Large amounts of blood may collect in the space between the galea and the skull, resulting in a subgaleal hematoma. Because infants have a smaller blood volume than adults, occasionally a young child may lose enough blood into a subgaleal hematoma to result in shock.

Mechanical factors also contribute to the severity and pattern of head injuries seen in pediatric patients. In childhood, the head is the largest part of the body mass, more than 25% in early infancy. Weak upper–extremity and neck muscles make it very difficult for a child to protect himself from head injury. In addition, the skull of the infant is very soft; as a result, a direct blow will easily deform the skull and may cause underlying cerebral injury. Fortunately, however, children have suture lines, which allow the skull to expand without causing compression of the brain. This enables the infant to suffer fewer effects from increased intracranial pressure for a short time.

PATHOPHYSIOLOGY

The brain, as a result of trauma, suffers both primary and secondary injury. Primary injury occurs as a direct result of the trauma (i.e., skull fractures, contusions, lacerations, and concussions). Once present, this damage is seldom influenced by therapeutic interventions.

Secondary injury occurs as a result of further brain insult from hypoxia (lack of oxygen), hypercapnea (lack of ventilation), or shock (lack of adequate perfusion to the brain). *Treatment of the head–injured child is aimed at preventing the secondary injury to improve outcome.*

Although many factors interact to determine the degree of secondary injury, the most crucial is increased intracranial pressure. Understanding the factors that influence intracranial pressure will aid the treatment of severe head trauma.

Cerebrospinal fluid, blood, and brain parenchyma are enclosed by the cranium. Constantly changing, the three attempt to maintain a relatively constant intracranial pressure. With an increase in the volume of one component, a decrease in one of the other two is necessary to maintain a constant, normal intracranial pressure, usually less than 15 mm Hg (Figure 8.2). Pulse, respiration, position changes, and Valsalva maneuvers also may cause some fluctuation in the intracranial pressure. When the brain is injured, the other intracranial components, cerebrospinal fluid and cerebral blood flow, attempt to buffer the system through compensation.

Cerebrospinal fluid contributes 10% of the total intracranial volume and is the first area affected when volume must be regulated. With an increase in intracranial volume, cerebrospinal fluid can be displaced easily into either the spinal subarachnoid space or the ventricular system to diminish cerebrospinal fluid volume. Both are attempts at maintaining the constant normal intracranial pressure. Marked changes in the intracranial pressure can occur with very small volume changes. When the cerebrospinal fluid shifts can no longer lessen the intracranial pressure, then cerebral blood flow attempts to lower pressure by altering flow.

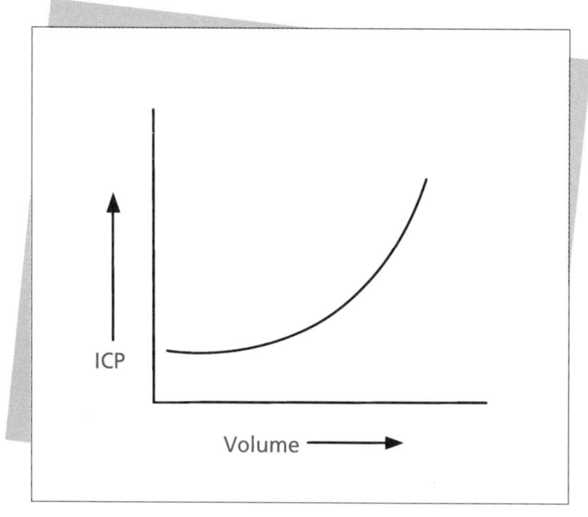

Figure 8.2. The correlation between increasing intracranial volume and increasing intracranial pressure.

Cerebral blood flow comprises only 8% of the intracranial volume, and changes in its volume can occur via several physiologic relationships. Thin–walled veins contain most of the cerebral blood volume, and with extrinsic tissue pressure, as occurs in cerebral edema, the cerebral veins attempt to compensate by decreasing their volume of cerebral blood. To assist a head-injured child with signs of impending herniation in keeping the intracranial pressure low, keep the head elevated and in the neutral midline position (using the backboard), hyperventilate the child, and keep the child well oxygenated, when possible.

Cerebral blood flow is also responsive to changes in carbon dioxide levels (Figure 8.3). Cerebral blood volume, and thus intracranial pressure, will decrease dramatically due to cerebral vasoconstriction, which is caused by rapidly lowering levels of carbon dioxide. Thus, hyperventilation of the child to prevent the accumulation of carbon dioxide will dramatically lower intracranial pressure. However, it will also lower intracranial perfussion and this is recommended only for the head-injured child with signs of impending herniation. Adequate oxygenation is also essential as hypoxia may lead to increased cerebral blood flow, increasing the intracranial pressure.

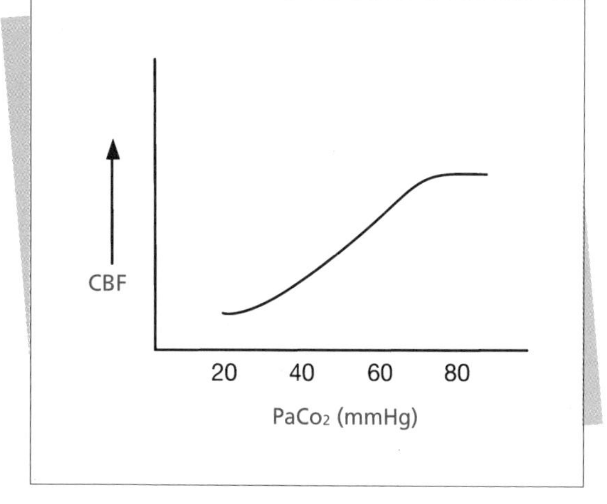

Figure 8.3. Association between increasing carbon dioxide levels and increasing cerebral blood flow.

The last 80% of the intracranial volume is made up by brain tissue. Obviously, with acute trauma there is little this mass can contribute to maintenance of a normal intracranial pressure.

ASSESSMENT

The assessment of the pediatric trauma patient begins with the arrival of the EMS personnel to the scene.

1. Scene survey
2. Airway, c–spine control, and initial LOC
3. Breathing
4. Circulation
5. Brief exam of abdomen, pelvis, and extremities
6. Critical transport decisions
7. Package and transport interventions
8. Secondary survey

Scene Survey

The mechanism of injury is particularly important to ascertain. In pediatric patients, it is also useful to note any clues of possible child abuse such as a chaotic home environment, discrepancies in caretakers' stories, or a reported mechanism of injury that does not fit with either the child's injuries or the patient's developmental age. Remember that an injured child may provoke extreme emotional responses from caretakers, ranging from anger to hysteria.

Historical information that must be obtained following a head injury includes loss of consciousness, amnesia for the event, severe headache, vomiting, and any change in the child's behavior. A short seizure immediately following a head injury is often benign but requires a complete medical assessment. All children who have had a head injury and then a seizure should be stabilized in the manner described below and transported. Any child with an altered mental status should be assumed to have a possible head injury and stabilized in the following manner.

Airway and C–spine

The initial approach to the patient should be made in a nonthreatening manner. Because the incidence of c–spine injuries in children with head trauma is high, it is particularly important to maintain c–spine immobilization in these patients. Any child with an altered mental status must have the c–spine immobilized. In an afebrile child with no history of a seizure disorder, prolonged seizure activity may be a sign of an occult head injury (shaken baby syndrome). Whenever uncertainty exists as to what has happened to the child, protect the c–spine.

Ensure that the patient has an open airway as manual control of the c–spine is taken. Sometimes children with head injuries will lose their gag reflex (will be unable to control their own secretions). Opening the airway via the modified jaw thrust maneuver and suctioning may be all that is needed for adequate airway control. In a child who is unconscious and has lost the gag reflex, an oropharyngeal airway may help to open the airway.

If the child is experiencing apneic episodes, immediately begin bag–valve–mask ventilations. To prevent the development of a secondary injury from hypoxia, the early administration of 100% oxygen is essential, even in conscious patients.

Breathing

Next, assess the child's respiratory status. It is important to keep in mind that irregular respirations are a sign of increased intracranial pressure. Be aggressive in assisting the child's ventilations if they aren't adequate. Hyperventilation is currently controversial in the management of head trauma. The patient should be ventilated at the normal respiratory rate for age unless there are obvious signs of herniation (unequal pupils). C–spine control should be continued with any manipulations of the airway.

Age	Weight in kg (lb)	Respirations	Pulse	Systolic Blood Pressure
Newborn	3–4 kg (6–9 lb)	30–50	120–160	60–80
6 mo–1 yr	8–10 kg (16–22 lb)	30–40	120–140	70–80
2–4 yr	12–16 kg (24–34 lb)	20–30	100–110	80–95
5–8 yr	18–26 kg (36–55 lb)	14–20	90–100	90–100
8–12 yr	26–50 kg (55–110 lb)	12–20	80–100	100–110
>12 yr	>50 kg (110 lb)	12–16	60–90	100–120

Table 8.1. Weight and vital signs by age group.

Circulation

After securing the airway and providing effective ventilations, assess the child's circulatory status. Shock rarely occurs following an isolated head injury, but it may be present with multisystem injury. Evaluation of the rate, rhythm, and quality of pulses, as well as the capillary refill, is necessary. Carefully stop all sites of active bleeding.

Bradycardia is an ominous sign and may be indicative of very high intracranial pressure. Cushing's Triad (bradycardia, hypertension, and irregular respirations) may be seen in children with very high intracranial pressure and indicates a severe head injury.

Because in children bradycardia also may occur with respiratory problems, *be sure that the airway is secure and give 100% oxygen.* Remember, maintaining ventilation and adequate oxygenation are vital.

Brief neurologic assessment. A child's level of consciousness may be assessed quickly by the AVPU system. A, alert; V, responds to verbal stimuli; P, responds to painful stimuli; and U, unresponsive. Another method for assessing the level of consciousness of a pediatric patient is the Glasgow Coma Scale modified for children (Table 8.2).

Using the Glasgow Coma Scale modified for children, any score less than 13 implies a serious head injury, and any score less than 7 is indicative of a profound, life–threatening neurologic dysfunction. *All children with an altered mental status require rapid package and transport.* The AVPU system is quicker and gives adequate information for making a decision on the severity of the head trauma in the field. If time is available, a Glasgow Coma Scale score should be obtained.

If a child continues to have seizures after a head injury, the patient must be managed carefully. Although a single short seizure following a head injury is usually benign, multiple seizures can be indicative of a severe head injury. Because seizures increase intracranial pressure, they need to be stopped as soon as possible. Follow local protocols, but remember that IV/IO or rectal diazepam or another benzodiazapine is usually effective.

	Patient > 2 yrs.	Patient < 2 yrs.	
Eye Opening	Spontaneous	Spontaneous	4
	To voice	To speech	3
	To pain	To pain	2
	None	None	1
Verbal Response	Oriented	Coos, babbles	5
	Confused	Cries irritably	4
	Inappropriate words	Cries to pain	3
	Incomprehensible	Moans to pain	2
	None	None	1
Motor Response	Obeys command	Normal movements	6
	Localizes pain	Withdraws - touch	5
	Withdrawal - pain	Withdrawal - pain	4
	Flexion - pain	Abnormal flexion	3
	Extension - pain	Abnormal extension	2
	None	None	1
Total : Eye + Verbal = Motor			

Table 8.2. Pediatric Glasgow Coma Scale.

Critical Transport Decisions

If any signs of an unstable airway, insufficient respirations, shock, or an altered mental status are present, the child should be packaged and transported rapidly.

Package and Transport Interventions

The key to a successful outcome following a head injury is early recognition and rapid management. Because head trauma accounts for 80% of pediatric trauma deaths, early, aggressive management will make a tremendous difference in the child's outcome.

If an object is impaled into the child's head, *do not remove it.* Stabilize the object in the position in which it is found.

During transport, lift the front of the backboard, if possible, so that the child's head is elevated. Ideally, the patient's head should also be kept in the midline position. Neither of these maneuvers is of high priority. *The most important issue is rapid transport to a center skilled in managing pediatric head trauma.*

Airway and c–spine. Complete c–spine immobilization should occur at this time. All children with an altered mental status require vigorous c–spine control to protect their spine during transport. If the child is not in shock and has an isolated head injury, the backboard or car seat head should be elevated 30 degrees to lower intracranial pressure.

All intubations should be performed en route to the hospital, if possible. Intubation attempts without the use of anesthetics may increase intracranial pressure. If a child is fighting the intubation attempt, effective bag–valve–mask ventilations should be performed en route to the hospital.

Obviously, airway control is best maintained by endotracheal intubation with in–line c–spine stabilization; however, this should be performed only by skilled personnel under controlled conditions to prevent further trauma and/or damage to the brain. Suctioning equipment should be easily accessible as emesis is a frequent problem in the head–injured child, particularly with manipulations of the airway.

Breathing. All head–injured children should receive 100% oxygen. If the child's ventilation is inadequate, it should be supported.

Circulation. If the child shows signs of shock, IV/IO access should be established and the standard 20 ml/kg bolus of normal saline administered. MAST trousers may be used as indicated (see Chapter 6). In order to maintain cerebral perfusion, the child must have an adequate circulating blood volume. It is critical to administer fluids to a child with head injury and shock.

In the absence of hemodynamic instability, IV access should be established and fluid administered at a rate to keep the vein open. If the MAST suit is applied in this situation, do not inflate as inflation of the trousers in a stable patient may increase intracranial pressure.

Secondary Survey

Head examination. During the examination of the head, look for signs of a serious injury. A careful examination of the head should reveal lacerations, hematomas, depressions, or cerebrospinal fluid leaks.

Note the depth and location of lacerations. Also note any fractures underneath a laceration. Carefully stop bleeding. Note the location and size of any swellings on the child's head. Be particularly careful if the hematoma is over the middle meningeal artery; some of these children may develop epidural bleeds. Depressions are easily palpable immediately following an injury. Note the depth and location. Note any fluid or blood draining from the nose or ears, Battle's sign, or raccoon eyes (Figure 8.4).

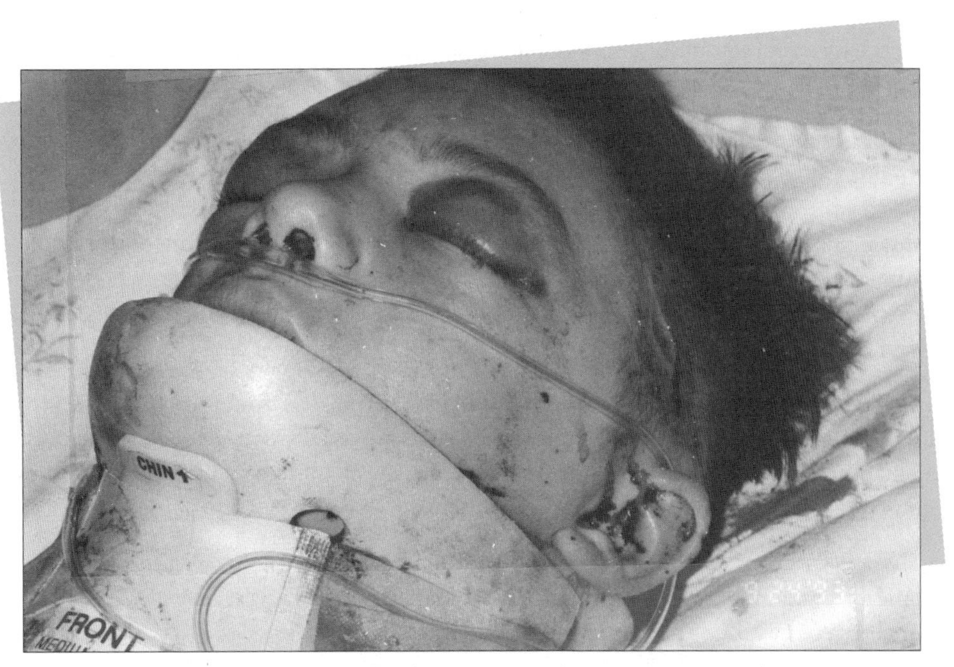

Figure 8.4. Patient with racoon eyes. (Intensive Care Unit)

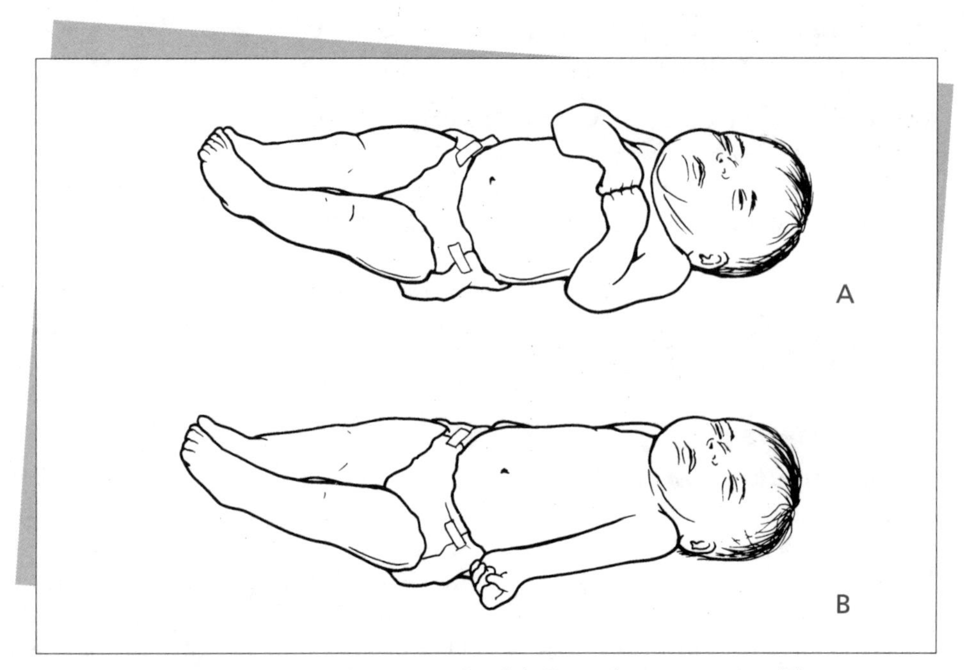

Figure 8.5. Decorticate posturing (A). Decerebrate posturing (B).

In children less than 1 year old, a fontanelle is present in the anterior portion of the skull. In infants, the fontanelle must be assessed, and while bulging or tenseness may be noted in a normal crying infant, any bulging in the quiet, upright baby may be indicative of increased intracranial pressure.

Complete neurologic examination. This examination should address the following areas.

Pupillary examination should note the size and reactivity of the pupils. Unequal or fixed and dilated pupils are indicative of severe trauma to the brain.

Motor and sensory examination should note the ability of the child to move the extremities. Check the motor strength and sensation in each extremity. In severe head injuries, a variety of abnormal muscle movements referred to as posturing may be noted. In decerebrate posturing, all extremities are extended and rotated inward (Figure 8.5). Decorticate posturing is recognized by the presence of extended legs and flexed arms (Figure 8.5). Progression from decorticate (flexion) posturing to decerebrate (extension) posturing is an ominous sign.

Careful reassessment is important in children with a head injury. With severe head trauma, the alterations in behavior and vital signs are usually present at the time of the initial evaluation. With mild–to–moderate head injuries, the changes may be ongoing, and early recognition and transport are critical in these patients.

Behavioral changes following a head injury may be progressive, subtle changes that indicate an internal injury. Information from parents or care givers may alert prehospital personnel to recent, subtle changes in the child's behavior. Always ask what the child is "normally" like.

Pharmacologic Management

Seizure medications – As mentioned earlier, seizures may occur with a head injury. Although most will be short and not cause complications, some severely head–injured children may have prolonged seizures that require aggressive therapy. These seizures, like any other in the pediatric population, may be treated with anticonvulsant medications along with the other interventions for head trauma (e.g., elevation of the head and hyperventilation).

Diuretics – Mannitol and furosemide may be used to release fluid from the child's body. This fluid loss also occurs from the brain, allowing the brain to "shrink" and cause a decrease in intracranial pressure. These medications work very effectively for an isolated head injury, especially in an intensive care unit, but are not reliable medications in the field.

Steroids – No study has shown steroids to be effective in the management of a head–injured patient; however, a single dose will not cause any problems.

TYPES OF HEAD INJURIES

Most pediatric head trauma involves extracranial injuries, such as lacerations and hematomas. Intracranial injuries are injuries to the brain that can cause serious morbidity and mortality. Other trauma that can occur to the skull, such as fractures, may be accompanied by an intracranial injury or, more commonly, occur as an isolated injury.

Extracranial Injuries

Lacerations and hematomas of the head are extremely common in children. All scalp lacerations should have a sterile dressing applied, and all active bleeding should be stopped in the primary survey. Note the location of all lacerations and hematomas because there may be a more serious injury, i.e., fracture or intracranial bleed, underneath.

Skull Fractures. There are three basic types of skull fractures: linear, depressed, and basilar.

Linear. Most linear skull fractures occur in young children and are fairly benign, unless accompanied by cerebral injury.

Depressed. Depressed skull fractures may be associated with blunt trauma, a penetrating object, or an overlying laceration, creating an open fracture. If a step–off or irregularity of the skull is palpable, avoid placing pressure on that area. If an object is present in the skull, stabilize it and do not attempt to remove it in the field. This type of fracture usually requires an operation to put the piece of bone into the correct location. Monitor these children closely because the brain may bleed where the skull pushes in on it.

Basilar. A basilar skull fracture is a clinical diagnosis. Signs associated with basilar skull fractures are cerebral spinal fluid leakage from either the ears or the nose, ecchymosis behind the ears (Battle's sign), and raccoon eyes (ecchymosis of the periorbital areas) (Figure 8.6). These fractures may involve the frontal, ethmoid, sphenoid, temporal, or occipital bones and may be quite serious. Sometimes the fracture will limit motion of the eyes and it may also be accompanied by cerebral injury. The biggest risk from these fractures is infection. With the cerebrospinal fluid communicating with the outside environment, bacteria can migrate into the fluid and cause infections such as meningitis.

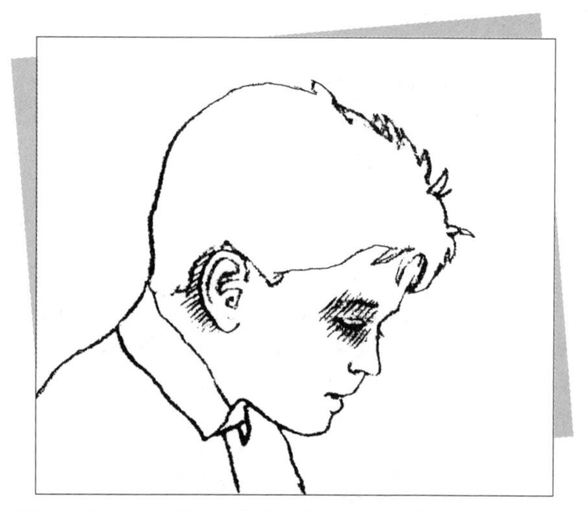

Figure 8.6. A child with Battle's sign and raccoon eyes.

Intracranial Injuries

Early identification of an intracranial injury is critical. These children need aggressive medical and surgical management to give them the best chance for a normal outcome.

Epidural hematomas. Beneath the skull lies the epidural space. This area is important because the meningeal arteries run through it, and, if they are damaged, severe hemorrhage can occur here. Fortunately, epidural hematomas are rare in children compared with adults. The most frequent cause of epidural hematoma is a temporal bone fracture that crosses the middle meningeal artery.

The usual presentation is a rapid deterioration of neurologic function with associated symptoms of increased intracranial pressure. These patients may have a subacute presentation or may be fine (lucid) following the injury, and then become progressively lethargic. That is why reassessment and monitoring of children with head trauma are so important.

Subdural hematomas. The dura mater, a fibrous layer that covers the brain, sits beneath the epidural space. Immediately below it is another layer, the arachnoid membrane. Between these layers run the meningeal veins. Subdural hematomas caused by bleeding from these veins are more common in children than epidural hematomas.

Because the bleeding is from veins instead of arteries, the onset of symptoms may take hours to days after the injury to develop. Symptoms, including lethargy, irritability, and either focal or generalized seizures, can be fairly nonspecific. These children also may have a bulging fontanelle, a sign of increased intracranial pressure, or retinal hemorrhages, a sign of abuse. It is important to keep in mind that subdural hemorrhages are often associated with shaken baby syndrome. This syndrome is a form of child abuse in which the infant is held and shaken; there usually are minimal signs of external injury, but the shaking results in serious brain injury.

Diffuse axonal injury. This is the most common type of injury with severe head trauma. The brain is injured so diffusely that there is diffuse subarachnoid blood and edema. The subarachnoid blood causes diffuse irritation that results in increased pressure and "leaking" of fluid into the brain. These patients also may have seizure activity and vomiting from the irritation.

Cerebral edema, or diffuse brain swelling, is the most difficult type of injury to manage. This swelling increases the intracranial pressure and may even lead to herniation, movement of brain tissue through the fibrous layers that surround the brain. Cushing's Triad (irregular respirations, bradycardia, and hypertension) is a sign of impending herniation, which is usually a terminating event for the brain. Herniation also may cause dilated, unreactive pupils, impairment of lateral or upward gaze, decreased level of consciousness, hypertonicity with decorticate or decerebrate posturing, and cardiorespiratory arrest.

Management is directed at decreasing the intracranial pressure through oxygenation, hyperventilation (this is the one indication for hyperventilation), and maintenance of blood flow to the brain.

Other Injuries

A cerebral hematoma is a collection of blood within the brain tissue. It is usually quite serious and the result of severe head trauma.

Other less severe forms of cerebral damage include contusions and concussions. Brain contusions are focal areas of swelling and bruising within the brain tissue. The neurologic findings are variable and depend on the location and extent of the bruising. Concussions represent a transient neurologic deficit secondary to trauma. This may include an altered level of consciousness, abnormal behavior, vomiting, headache, or amnesia that improves over time. Early in their course, concussions cannot be differentiated from intracranial injury; all children with these symptoms need a complete medical evaluation and continuous monitoring.

Points to Remember

1. Head trauma is the leading cause of traumatic death in the pediatric population.
2. The large size of the head and weak neck muscles predispose children to serious head injury.
3. Careful assessment and appropriate interventions such as oxygenation, hyperventilation, and maintenance of cerebral blood flow are necessary to prevent secondary brain injury and to control intracranial pressure.
4. All serious head injuries should be considered life–threatening and require aggressive management of the ABCs.
5. Any child with an altered mental status should be rapidly packaged and transported to the nearest appropriate facility.

Bibliography

1. Ackerman AD: Current issues in the care of the head injured child. *Curr Opin Pediatr* 1991;3:433–438.
2. American Academy of Pediatrics, American College of Emergency Physicians (1989) APLS:The Pediatric Emergency Medicine Course, First edition. 95–111.
3. Bouma GJ, et al: Blood pressure and intracranial pressure–volume dynamics in severe head injury. *J Neurosurg* 1992;77:15–19.
4. Bruce DA, et al: Diffuse cerebral swelling following head injuries in children. *J Neurosurg* 1992;54:170–178.
5. Dean JM: Cerebral protection and neurologic outcome following closed head injury in children. *Curr Opin Pediatr* 1990;2:514–518.
6. Ghajar J, Hariri RJ: Management of pediatric head injury. *Pediatr Clin North America* 1992;39:1093–1125.
7. Inaba AS, Seward PN: An approach to pediatric trauma. *Emerg Med Clin North America* 1991;9:523–548.
8. Johnston MV, Gerring JP: Head trauma and its sequelae. *Pediatr Ann* Vol 21:362– 368.
9. Mayer TA, Walker ML: Pediatric head injury. *Ann Emerg Med* 1985;14:1178–1184.
10. Nichols DG, Yaster M, Lappe DG, et al: (1991) Golden Hour The Handbook of Pediatric Life Support, St Louis, MO: The CV Mosby Co., 289–309.
11. Simon JE, Goldberg AT. (1989) *Prehospital Pediatric Life Support,* St Louis, MO: The CV Mosby Co. 42–49, 70–81.

Pediatric Extremity Trauma

Janet H. Metzger, RN
Ronald R. McWilliams, NREMT–P

Introduction

Injuries to the musculoskeletal system in children are common and usually are not life–threatening. Extremity injuries, however, may be accompanied by other injuries. The priority of care in any traumatic setting is to treat life–threatening injuries first. The goals for treating children with extremity trauma are to *stabilize the patient, prevent further injuries, and maximize the functional outcome from the trauma.*

ANATOMY/PHYSIOLOGY

Children have specific anatomic and physiologic properties inherent to their bones that contribute to unique injury patterns. The following are features of pediatric bones: the presence of epiphyses (growth plates), which in children are a frequent site of injury (growth disturbances may result from these injuries); incomplete fractures, which commonly occur in children's bones because of their resilience and elasticity; and rapid healing.

Other injuries, such as dislocations and compartment syndromes, are not commonly seen in children. Sprains and strains occur frequently in the pediatric population, but in the field these can be very difficult to differentiate from a fracture.

ASSESSMENT

Assessment is of primary importance in the management of any patient; even if an isolated extremity injury is suspected, the entire primary and secondary survey must be performed.

1. Scene survey
2. Airway, c–spine control, and initial LOC
3. Breathing
4. Circulation
5. Brief exam of abdomen, pelvis, and extremities
6. Critical transport decisions
7. Package and transport interventions
8. Secondary survey

Scene Survey

The mechanism of injury contributes significantly to the management of a child with extremity trauma. Significant force is required to cause certain fractures in children and may cause multisystem injury in a young patient. Eighty to 90% of childhood injuries are caused by blunt trauma.[1] Preventable trauma accounts for 25% of fractures in children less than 3 years old.[2] Mechanisms likely to cause localized musculoskeletal injuries include lawn mower accidents, farm equipment injuries, and bicycle accidents.

Airway and C–spine

Because patients with extremity injuries often have multisystem injury, carefully secure the c–spine. Assess and manage the airway as discussed in Chapter 4.

Breathing

When children are in pain, they may become tachypneic (breathe fast). They should receive 100% oxygen and be monitored very closely. If other injuries are identified, these should be managed as indicated in earlier chapters.

Circulation

As indicated in Chapter 6, even small amounts of blood loss may result in shock in a child. Tachycardia and poor perfusion indicate possible shock. Carefully stop all active sites of bleeding.

If the child has an amputation, immediate care should be focused on the stump. Stump care is aimed at controlling bleeding by application of a pressure dressing. If the injury involves a major extremity, the bleeding may be excessive and result in shock; therefore, early application of a dressing will minimize blood loss.

Critical Transport Decisions

All children with evidence of shock should be transported immediately. In addition, rapid transport is indicated for any child with an amputation of a major extremity.

Package and Transport Interventions

Airway and c–spine. Provide care as discussed in Chapters 4 and 7.

Breathing. Provide care as discussed in Chapter 5.

Circulation. Provide care as discussed in Chapter 6. A rapid trauma survey should be performed initially, and military antishock trousers may be used to stabilize any lower–extremity fracture or possible pelvic fracture. Pelvic or femur fractures may result in substantial blood loss. All IV access should be obtained en route to the hospital.

Secondary Survey

Extremity assessment. The extremity assessment is part of the secondary survey. If a child is unstable, the secondary survey should be performed en route to the hospital. In some critically injured children, an extremity assessment may not occur in the field. As mentioned previously, the only time the extremity assessment should be part of the primary survey is if active bleeding is present from the injury or as part of the rapid trauma survey. Rapid application of a pressure dressing may prevent shock from developing and minimize ongoing fluid losses.

During the assessment of an extremity injury, the following items should be checked: soft tissue for ecchymosis, breaks in the continuity of the skin, tenderness, and swelling; motor function (Is the patient able to move the extremity on command?); sensory function (Does the patient respond to touch, pain, etc. in the extremity?); and circulation for pulses; skin temperature, moisture, and color; and capillary refill.

Document the initial findings and carefully monitor the child for changes during transport. Document sensation, motor function, and circulation before and after the application of a splint.

FRACTURES/DISLOCATIONS

The bones of pediatric patients have unique anatomic and physiologic properties that account for the large number of fractures that occur during childhood.

Most pediatric fractures are classified in a manner similar to that for adults. Decide whether the fracture is open or closed. Open fractures have a laceration over the site of trauma. They are more likely to become infected because of contamination. Therefore, it is important that all lacerations and open areas are noted prior to the application of a dressing. Most fractures in children are simple fractures (the bone is broken into two pieces) and not comminuted (the bone is broken into multiple pieces).

Two unique fractures of childhood are the greenstick fracture (Figure 9.1), which results when a bone breaks on the outer surface but is maintained intact on its inner surface, and the torus fracture (Figure 9.2), which is caused by buckling of the outer surface.

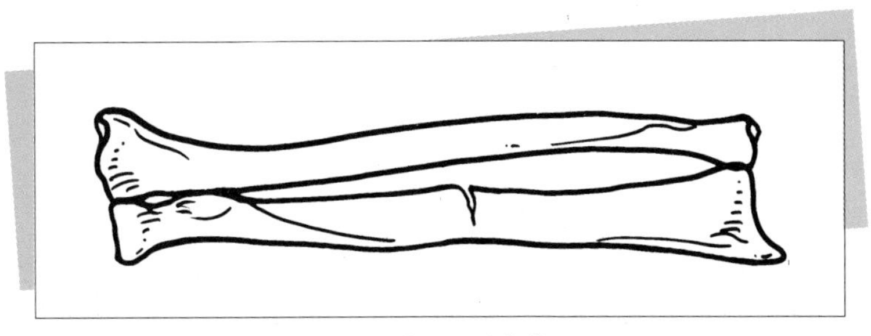

Figure 9.1. Greenstick fracture.

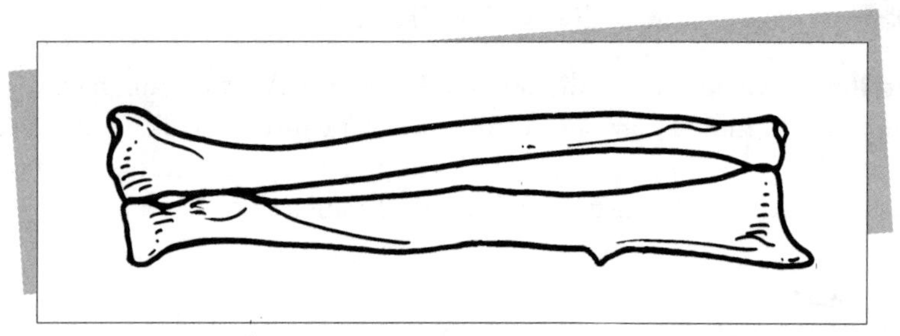

Figure 9.2. Torus fracture.

Although dislocations occur infrequently in children, they can be a major cause of morbidity. It is important to check the neurovascular function below any joint that is swollen or painful.

Signs and Symptoms

In general, children with fractures should be assessed in the same way as adults. Usually the child will have pain, swelling, and deformity at the site of the injury. If there is uncertainty as to whether a fracture exists, *treat the injury as a fracture.* If the fracture involves a joint, there also may be decreased range of motion and possible vascular compromise.

Treatment

The goals of fracture management include stabilization, reduction of pain, and prevention of further injury. To accomplish these goals, proper equipment must be available and the provider should be very familiar with immobilization techniques. Inappropriate immobilization may result in loss of function in the extremity and serious long–term problems for the child.

In the stabilization of a fracture or suspected fracture, not only must the actual injury site be immobilized, but the joint above and the joint below the injury must be immobilized as well. If there is a break in the continuity of the soft tissue, a sterile pressure dressing must be applied.

Once the bleeding is controlled and the extremity is appropriately bandaged, to immobilize the injury. *Always check the pulse, motor, and sensory functions of the extremity before and after immobilization.* Document findings.

If a child has a dislocation, immobilize it in a position in which the patient is most comfortable and the neurovascular status is intact. Transport to the nearest facility.

Specific Extremity Treatments.

Shoulder – Sling and swathe. Elbow should be flexed at a 90–degree angle with some support between the elbow and the abdomen.

Elbow – Immobilization in position found. *Do not* manipulate as severe neurovascular complications may occur. Sling and swathe when possible.

Wrist – Board splint with gauze placed between fingers, and support hand on board with roller gauze on palmar side of hand. Apply ice and elevate above the level of the chest.

Hip – Immobilize in position found. Secure to backboard.

Knee – Immobilize in position found. If distal pulse is absent, apply gentle longitudinal traction to the limb. Secure to backboard.

Ankle – Splint in position of injury using pressure.

Foot – Dressing (pillow–type splint). Apply ice and elevate extremity above chest level if possible.

Humerus – Rigid–type splint to immobilize the fracture site. Sling and swathe.

Forearm – Rigid–type splint to immobilize the fracture site. Sling and swathe.

Hand – Rigid–type splint with gauze placed between fingers. Support hand on board with roller gauze on ventral side. Apply ice and elevate above the level of the chest.

Pelvis – Splint with military antishock trousers. Watch abdominal inflation, which may cause respiratory compromise. Following military antishock trouser inflation, or if the trousers are not available, secure to backboard.

Femur – If a femur fracture is present, apply a traction splint (Figure 9.3) or military antishock trousers. If a fracture is assessed at distal end (pain above knee, deformity, instability, and angulation of thigh), use rigid–type splint. Secure to backboard.

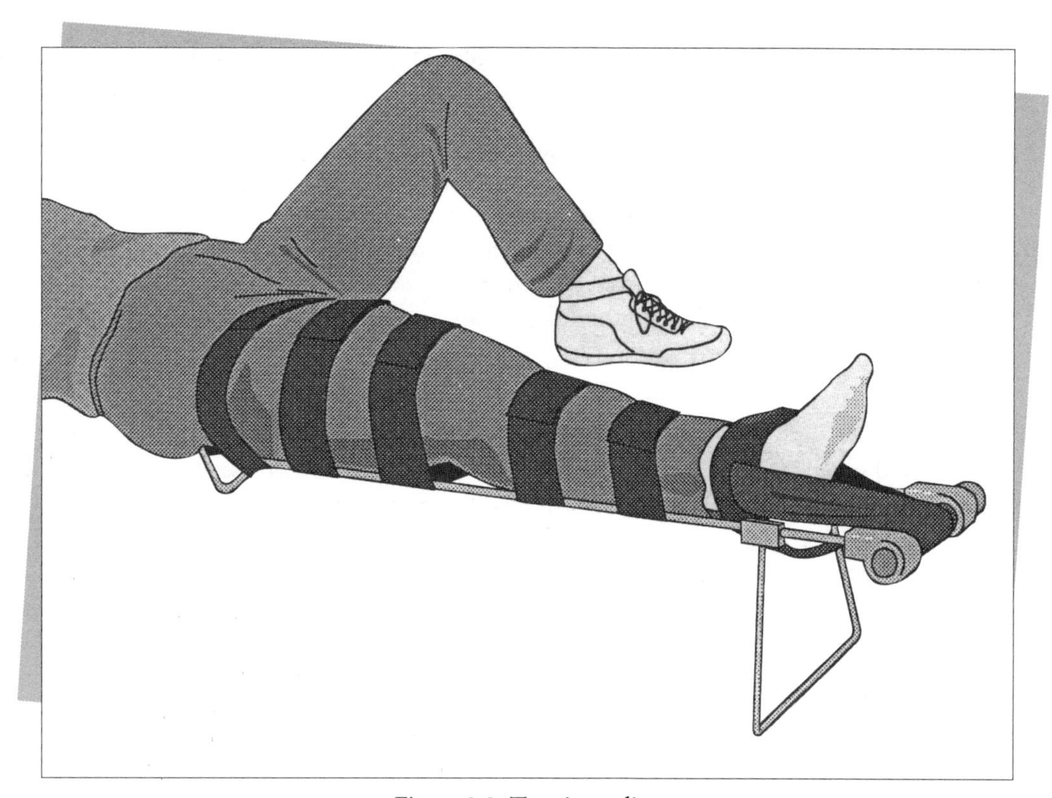

Figure 9.3. Traction splint.

Tibia/Fibula – Rigid–type splint and secure to backboard.

Ankle/Foot – Splint using pressure dressing (pillow–type splint). Apply ice and elevate extremity above chest level if possible.

Splinting of an extremity should not be taken lightly, even though it is a basic skill. Several complications, including changing a closed fracture to an open fracture, causing neurovascular compromise, and creating a greater displacement of a joint, may occur if done improperly.

Not all trauma patients will or should be splinted as previously described. In the multisystem trauma patient (see Package and Transport Interventions), splinting may be best accomplished by using the body and backboard as the only splint. Remember that the ABCs should always take priority over the extremities.

SPRAINS/STRAINS

Sprains are ligamentous injuries that occur about the joint. Strains are tears of the muscle tendon junction and usually occur away from joints.[2]

Signs and Symptoms

In the field, these injuries are not easily differentiated from fractures, with most of the children presenting with pain and swelling.

Treatment

The initial treatment of a sprain or strain will follow fracture management principles.

COMPARTMENT SYNDROME

A compartment syndrome results from increased pressure within a closed space, as a result of blunt or penetrating trauma. Compartment syndromes have many causes, including tight dressings, splints, or casts; or internal bleeding or edema following an injury.[3] Early recognition of this syndrome is crucial in preventing permanent nerve and vascular damage to the extremity.

Signs and Symptoms

Signs and symptoms of this syndrome are severe pain, muscle weakness, numbness, and swelling of the extremity. Pulses may be present initially and then gradually disappear. *The loss of the pulse is a very late finding.*

Treatment

If unrecognized, a compartment syndrome can lead to permanent loss of function in the extremity. Splint the extremity and notify the receiving facility of the possibility of a compartment syndrome. A skilled surgeon will need to release the pressure (through fasciotomy) as quickly as possible to preserve function.

AMPUTATIONS

Amputations are either complete or incomplete. The mechanisms causing an amputation are clean–cut injury (guillotine–type), crush injury, or avulsion injury. The repair of an incomplete amputation is known as *revascularization*. The repair or reattachment of a completely amputated part is known as *replantation*.

A clean–cut amputation has the best rate of successful repair after microsurgery. The success rate for digital replants is less in children, but when they succeed, the function is better than in adults.[4] The small size of the vessels in children makes the repair of these technically difficult. The decision about treatment is made after many considerations when an amputation injury has occurred. The hand dominance, importance of the part for function, associated injuries, and nature of the injury are all taken into consideration.

Signs and Symptoms

Identify all areas of potential injury. Determine whether the amputation is partial or complete. If the child had active bleeding from the site, this determination will have been made in the circulation portion of the assessment.

Treatment

The goals of treatment include control of bleeding and preservation of amputated parts. Although individual facilities will have specific protocols for managing amputations, the following information should serve as a guideline for the care of both complete and incomplete amputations.

Complete Amputations

Care of the stump is addressed in the circulation portion of the assessment. Be sure to control the bleeding through the application of a pressure dressing. Always take care of the stump before caring for the amputated part. Amputated parts should be retrieved and rinsed with sterile saline or lactated Ringer's solution. This removes gross contaminants. The part should be wrapped in a *saline–moistened* (*not* soaked) gauze and placed in a plastic bag or container and *sealed*. The sealed container should be placed in another container with ice. The tissue should never contact the ice. *Never use dry ice*. The proper cooling of amputated parts slows metabolism and extends ischemic time, allowing the surgeon time for microsurgical repair or reconstruction.[5]

Incomplete Amputations

Treatment of incomplete amputations will be similar to that of complete amputations. Control bleeding, then place a moist saline or lactated Ringer's dressing over open tissue. Apply a pressure dressing and splint, if necessary, to stop the bleeding and stabilize the injury. Place ice packs over the area without blood flow. Place ice over a dressing, *never directly on the skin*.

Points to Remember

1. Extremity injuries are extremely common in children.
2. Always begin with the assessment and stabilize the ABCs first.
3. All extremity injuries should be stabilized, if time allows, for reduction of pain and to prevent further injury.

Bibliography

1. Stellar J: *Pediatrics, A Comprehensive Curriculum for Trauma Nursing.* Boston, Jones and Bartlett Publishers, 1992.
2. Barkin R, Rosen P: *Management Principles, Emergency Pediatrics,* ed 3. St Louis, CV Mosby Co, 1990, p 418–429.
3. Reff RB: *Musculoskeletal Injury, Pediatric Trauma Care.* Rockville, Maryland, Aspen Publishers, Inc, 1988, p 133–144.
4. Cmiel P, Cavanaugh CE: Digital replantation in children. *Am J Nursing* 1989;9:1158–1161.
5. Richards RR, Urbaniak JR: The surgical and rehabilitation management of vascular injury to the hand. *Hand Clinics.* 1986;2:171–177.

Suggested Reading

1. Eichelberger M, Stossel–Pratsch G: *Pediatric Emergencies Manual.* Rockville, Maryland, Aspen Publishers, Inc, 1984, p 76–86.
2. Gazzaniga AB, Iseri LT, Baren M: *Emergency Care: Principles and Practices for the EMT–Paramedic.* Reston, Virginia, Reston Publishing Co, Inc., 1979, p 417–429.
3. Ogden JA: The uniqueness of growing bones, in *Fractures in Children,* ed 3. Philadelphia, JB Lippincott Co, 1991.
4. Schultz RJ: *The Language of Fractures,* ed 2. Baltimore, Williams & Wilkins, 1990, p 36–45.
5. Simon JE, Goldberg AT: *Prehospital Pediatric Life Support.* St Louis, CV Mosby Co, 1990, p 78–81.

Pediatric Abdominal Trauma

Sharon Deppe, RN
Bonnie Beaver, MD, FACS,FAAP

Introduction

Blunt trauma accounts for the majority of abdominal injuries in children. Significant intra–abdominal trauma occurs in 25% of multisystem injuries.[1] The most common mechanism of injury for the pediatric multiple–trauma patient is described as a motor vehicle crash with the child being a pedestrian. This usual triad of injury (Waddell's Triad) involves the head, trunk, and extremity. Other predominant sources of injury include falls, direct blows to the abdomen, incorrectly worn lap belt restraint devices, bicycle collisions, and child abuse.

It is often difficult to recognize when a child has sustained an injury to the abdomen. Patient anxiety, the comfort level of the health care provider, and the child's limited communication skills may affect the ability to discover subtle changes that warrant immediate intervention and further evaluation. Undetected, abdominal trauma in the pediatric patient can lead to shock and death.

Through a brief and accurate systematic assessment, appropriate intervention, and rapid transport, the child with abdominal trauma can have an excellent outcome. Children with penetrating injuries to the abdomen, while not as common (5%),[1] can also have a positive outcome if managed appropriately.

ANATOMY/PATHOPHYSIOLOGY

The child's abdomen can be divided into four quadrants. Located below the diaphragm, the abdominal cavity contains both solid and hollow organs. Blunt trauma to any of the quadrants can cause a rupture or tear of an organ.

The spleen is a blood–filled organ located in the left upper quadrant and partially protected by the lower ribs. Despite this protection, it is the most commonly injured organ. Blunt force can cause the spleen to fracture or shatter (occurs more commonly) or become lacerated by a fractured rib (occurs less commonly).

The liver is a solid, vascular organ in the right upper quadrant located under the right lower rib cage. While less commonly injured than the spleen,[2] rupture or laceration of the liver can cause severe hemorrhage. Injury to the liver is the most common abdominal injury that leads to death.

The true abdomen (right and left lower quadrants) contains the large and small intestines and the bladder. Damage to these organs can result in infection and shock.

Behind the true abdomen lies the retroperitoneal space containing the kidneys, ureters, pancreas, duodenum, abdominal aorta, and inferior vena cava. A child's kidney is more vulnerable to blunt injury than an adult's because it is proportionately larger and less protected by bone and muscle.[3] While relatively encased by other organs in the retroperitoneal space, the pancreas and duodenum are injured less often than other organs but can have serious consequences when involved.

Pediatric abdominal muscles are less developed than those of adults and, therefore, less defined. This accounts for the "pot–bellied" appearance that infants and toddlers exhibit when lying or standing. This thinner muscle wall should make the pediatric abdomen easier to assess than that of the adult, but anxiety and pain can cause a child to cry, causing muscles to tighten and make abdominal assessment more difficult. The air swallowed while crying can also distort the abdomen, making it appear more distended; this causes increased discomfort and may impair respiratory effort by displacing the diaphragm into the thorax. Any positive–pressure ventilation may also result in abdominal distention.

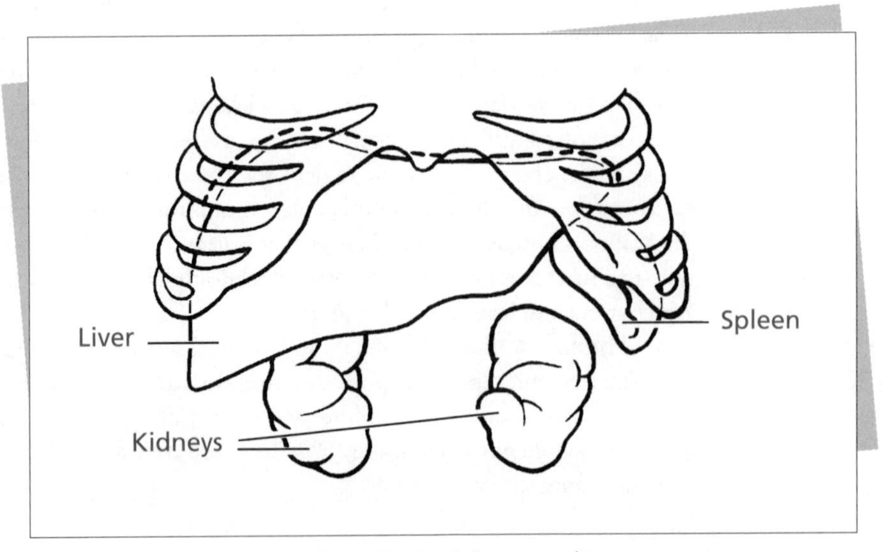

Figure 10.1. The pediatric abdomen and its contents.

ASSESSMENT

Determining the mechanism of injury becomes vital when evaluating the pediatric patient. This information can alert the health care provider to injury potential, as discussed in Chapter 2. Blunt trauma often exhibits minimal external signs, and the infant or young child cannot assist the examiner by describing the pain.

In general, the following scheme should be followed:

1. Scene survey
2. Airway, c–spine control, and initial LOC
3. Breathing
4. Circulation
5. Brief exam of abdomen, pelvis, and extremities
6. Critical transport decisions
7. Package and transport interventions
8. Secondary survey

Scene Survey

At the scene, it is important to note the circumstances surrounding the traumatic event. If the child is involved in a motor vehicle collision, observations related to speed of vehicle, extent of damage, account of any extrication procedures, distance thrown or ejected, surface or object of contact, and use of shoulder or lap belt warrant a high index of suspicion for multisystem injury with potential abdominal involvement.

Airway and C–spine

Because abdominal trauma is usually associated with injury to other systems, initial assessment begins with the ABCs.

Stabilize the patient's c–spine and manage the airway as discussed in Chapter 4. Any patient suspected of having an abdominal injury should be placed on 100% oxygen.

Breathing

Assessment of the child's breathing should be performed next. Use the protocol discussed in Chapters 4 and 5 to recognize a child in respiratory distress or failure and manage appropriately. When internal bleeding is present, the normally soft, round pediatric abdomen becomes rigid, distended, and guarded. The child's respiratory effort is marked by expiratory grunting in an attempt to splint pain and increase force on the diaphragm for improved exhalation. Large amounts of blood in the abdomen can impair ventilation as the accumulation of fluid begins to restrict diaphragmatic movement. Blood and bile are irritants to the diaphragm, and the presence of either can be exhibited as referred pain. Injury to the spleen or liver can produce pain to the left shoulder (Kehr's Sign) through diaphragmatic irritation.

Circulation

Many children with intra–abdominal injuries will present with signs and symptoms suggestive of shock. As indicated earlier, tachycardia can be an early sign of intra–abdominal bleeding. The heart rate increases in an attempt to circulate blood and maintain blood pressure. Tachycardia continues until cardiac reserve is depleted and the blood pressure drops. *Hypotension is a late and ominous sign of hypovolemia.*[4] During the initial assessment all external sources of bleeding should be stopped with dressings.

EXAMINE THE ABDOMEN, PELVIS, AND EXTREMITIES (QUICK SURVEY)

Brief Neurological Assessment

Because children with abdominal injuries will usually have other injuries, perform a careful neurologic assessment as discussed in previous chapters. As with adults, abdominal pain may not be easily assessed in the child with a decreased level of consciousness.

Critical Transport Decisions

Many pediatric patients with a significant abdominal injury will show signs of shock. Any pediatric patient who exhibits signs of shock should be packaged and transported immediately. In addition, any child who has an accompanying unstable airway, respiratory insufficiency, or altered mental status should be packaged and transported as quickly as possible. A child with potential abdominal injury should be secured to a backboard. An infant or toddler in a car seat should be removed from it. Because the extent of internal injury will be unknown, immobilization of the abdomen and pelvis can help limit further injury and internal hemorrhage.

PACKAGE AND TRANSPORT INTERVENTIONS

Airway and c-spine. Provide care as discussed in Chapters 4 and 7.

Breathing. As discussed in previous chapters, make sure the child is placed on 100% oxygen. It is important to keep a child with an abdominal injury well oxygenated.

Circulation. Military antishock trousers, while controversial, may be considered as a temporary intervention for the pediatric patient in extreme shock or with known extremity fractures. Inflate the leg compartments to control extremity bleeding and splint fractures. Inflation of the abdominal compartment may cause the abdominal contents to restrict diaphragmatic movement and cause respiratory distress. Deflation of the military antishock trousers should be done only in the hospital after adequate fluid resuscitation.

Procedures, when possible, should be performed en route to the hospital. If a child is in shock, venous access may be attempted en route for fluid resuscitation. Fluid boluses of lactated Ringer's or normal saline should be given to increase circulating volume (see Chapter 6). The child who continues to be hemodynamically unstable and has failed to respond to aggressive fluid resuscitation may require emergency surgery and should be transported rapidly to a pediatric facility.

Orogastric tube insertion. At some time during the stabilization of a child with abdominal trauma, an orogastric tube should be inserted. If the child's respiratory status is compromised from abdominal distention, this may be performed in the field. If time is not available or protocols do not allow, it may be performed electively on arrival in the emergency department. The correct positioning of the tube is important to insure proper function.

Secondary Survey

Abdominal examination. With the child's clothing removed, conduct a rapid assessment of the abdomen. Inspect the skin for ecchymosis, abrasions, and marks. Bruising to the umbilicus, flank, scrotum, or labia indicates potential internal bleeding. Pain and linear markings over the chest and abdomen and low back pain can be an indication of a shoulder–lap belt injury. Rib fractures, intestinal perforations, and lumbar compression fractures have been associated with "seatbelt syndrome" injuries.[5,6]

Physical Signs and Symptoms Suggestive of Abdominal Trauma
▪ Pain
▪ Tenderness
▪ Distention
▪ Peritoneal signs
▪ Bruises
▪ Tire tracks
▪ Seat-belt marks
▪ Kehr's sign: pain in the left should induced by palpation of LUQ
▪ Turner's sign: ecchymotic discoloration of the flank
▪ Cullen's sign: ecchymotic discoloration of the umbilicus
▪ Unexplained hypotension or other signs of hypovolemic shock

Table 10.1. Physical signs and symptoms suggestive of abdominal trauma.

The recent pediatric literature has demonstrated that most blunt abdominal injuries in children can be managed conservatively with fluid therapy and close observation.[7] Children receive a computed tomography (CT) scan of their abdomen to delineate internal injuries. If the volume deficit cannot be corrected or there is evidence of persistent bleeding, the child may be taken to the operating room. This conservative approach has led to a drastic reduction in the morbidity and mortality associated with abdominal injuries.

Penetrating trauma. If there is evidence of a penetrating injury on physical examination, treatment is the same as for an adult. Any object that protrudes from the abdomen should not be removed. Reinforcing the object to the body with a stabilizing, bulky dressing can help prevent further damage.

If entrance and exit wounds are visible, they signal a penetrating traumatic injury. Occasionally, only an entrance wound may be seen. The extent of injury may not be determined by the location of the entrance wound. A bullet may pass erratically through many organs in an irregular course. If penetrating trauma occurs to the lower–chest area, the abdomen should also be assessed for involvement. Penetrating injury to the abdominal wall can cause internal contents to protrude to the outside. These evisceration injuries should be covered with a moist, sterile saline dressing. Do not attempt to return the visible organ back into the abdominal cavity. *Never inflate military antishock trousers over an eviscerated bowel.*

Points to Remember

1. Because most pediatric abdominal injuries are subtle, a high degree of suspicion must be maintained.
2. Perform a rapid, systematic assessment.
3. Patients exhibiting signs of shock are "rapid package and transport" situations. Procedures should be performed en route to the hospital.

Bibliography

1. Newman KD, Eichelberger MR, Randolph JG: Abdominal trauma, in Eichelberger MR (ed): *Pediatric Trauma Care.* Rockville, Maryland, Aspen Publishers, Inc., 1988, p101– 102.
2. Marx JA: Abdominal trauma, in Barkin RM, Rosen P (eds): *Emergency Pediatrics; A Guide to Ambulatory Care.* St Louis, CV Mosby Co, 1990, p 397.
3. Kass EJ: Genitourinary injury, in Eichelberger MR (ed): *Pediatric Trauma Care.* Rockville, Maryland, Aspen Publishers, Inc, 1988, p105.
4. Chameides L (ed): *Textbook of Pediatric Advanced Life Support.* Dallas, American Heart Association, 1990.
5. Tso E, Beaver B, Haller A: Abdominal injuries in restrained pediatric passengers. *J of Ped Surg* 1993;7:915–919.
6. Reid AB, Letts RM, Black GB: Pediatric chance fractures: Association with intra–abdominal injuries and seat belt use. *J Trauma* 1990;30:384–391.
7. Galat JA, Grisone ER, Gauderer M: Pediatric blunt liver injury: Establishment of criteria for appropriate management. *J Pediatr Surg* 1990;25:1162–1165.
8. Eichelberger MR, Zwick HA, et al: Pediatric trauma protocol: A team approach, in Eichelberger MR (ed): *Pediatric Trauma Care.* Rockville, Maryland, Aspen Publishers, Inc, 1988, p 15.

Pediatric Burns

Howard A. Werman, MD, FACEP

Introduction

Each year in the United States, two million people seek medical attention for treatment of burns, and 100,000 people are hospitalized. Nearly half of these injuries occur in pediatric patients. Children less than 3 years old have the greatest risk of long–term morbidity and mortality among burn victims.

The majority of burns in children are caused by thermal injuries. In children less than 3 years old, scald burns (from hot liquids) are the most common cause of burns, whereas the incidence of flame burns increases after the age of 2 years. Electrical, lightning, and chemical injuries are much less common in children.

The health care provider must remember several important points in caring for the pediatric burn victim. The first priority should be to *safely* remove the victim from the source of injury (fire, smoke, electricity, chemicals, etc.). Remember that although burns can be quite dramatic in appearance, attention must first be focused on the child's airway, breathing, and circulation. Life–threatening injuries can develop in children with burns as the result of trauma from automobile collisions, falls from heights, or blast injuries. Finally, aggressive resuscitation in the early phases of burn injury can improve the child's long–term prospects for a full recovery.

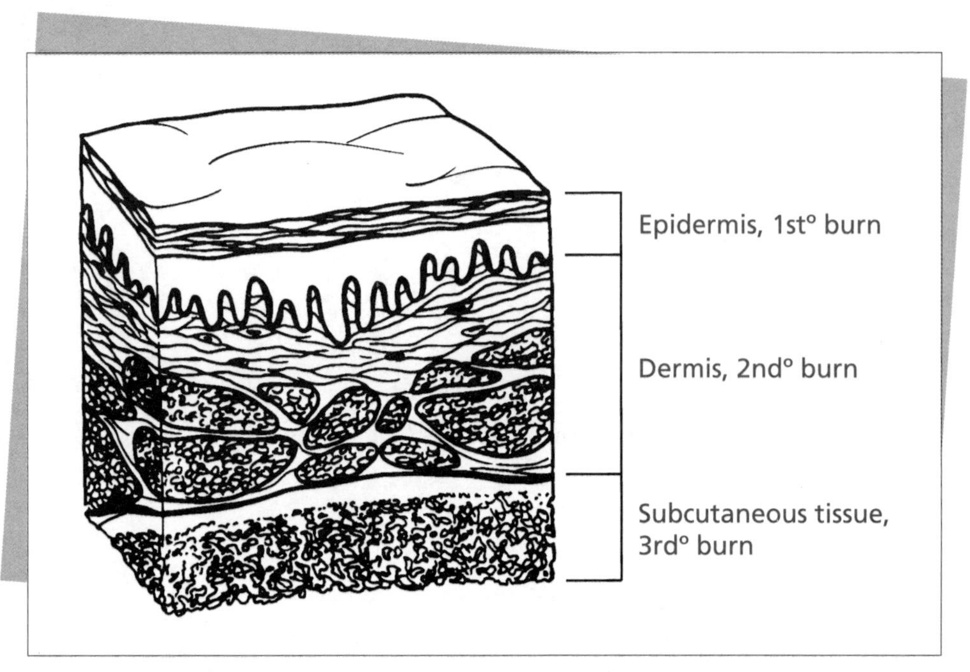

Figure 11.1. The epidermis, dermis, and subqutaneous tissue.

ANATOMY/PHYSIOLOGY

Burns are caused by the application of heat to the skin and underlying structures. The skin is divided into two layers: the epidermis and dermis (Figure 11.1). The epidermis is the most superficial area of the skin and consists of several thick layers of cells. The primary function of the epidermis is to protect the body against invasion from microorganisms and to prevent leakage of body fluids. The dermis is a connective tissue layer that lies beneath the epidermis. It contains several important skin appendages, including hair follicles, sweat glands, nerve endings, and blood vessels. The dermis is crucial for several important skin functions, including temperature regulation and regeneration of damaged skin.

Inhalation Injury

Inhalation injury occurs when heated air, smoke, and toxic products of combustion are inhaled from a heat source. Children with inhalation injury can have serious airway and pulmonary complications, often without any external signs of significant burn. Half of the deaths from burns are the result of inhalation injury.

The effects of the inhalation are caused by the direct effect of heat on the airway and bronchial tree (airway obstruction and wheezing) as well as toxic effects of smoke, carbon monoxide, and cyanide. Carbon monoxide is an odorless, colorless byproduct of incomplete combustion of many common compounds. Carbon monoxide prevents the binding of oxygen on hemoglobin in the bloodstream and prevents oxygen from being used efficiently by cells. Cyanide acts in a similar fashion. Recent studies have shown that cyanide is often found in toxic levels in patients with significant inhalation injury.

High–Voltage Electrical Injuries

These injuries present with a very different clinical picture. The burns from the entrance and exit of current are often unimpressive, unless the child's clothing was ignited. However, there is often extensive damage of the nerves, blood vessels, and muscles in the path of current through the child's body. Damage to the heart can cause cardiogenic shock and arrhythmias, especially ventricular fibrillation. In addition, release of myoglobin from damaged muscle can deposit in the kidneys and cause long–term renal failure if not treated aggressively. High–voltage electricity injuries are often accompanied by violent contraction of the skeletal muscles, leading to fractures and dislocations involving the long bones and spine. In addition, other injuries can result when the child falls following contact with a high–voltage wire.

The most common electrical burns in children involve oral burns that occur after a child bites into a live electrical wire. Although bodily injury is unlikely, the child requires a careful evaluation with particular attention to the extent of oral damage.

Lightening Injuries

Lightening injuries are also seen in children. Although these injuries involve high–voltage electricity, they produce much higher currents (10,000,000 to 2,000,000,000 V) over a very brief period (milliseconds). Such injuries result in little internal injury and few surface burns. Instead, the majority of these patients present with profound respiratory arrest that leads to asystole. These patients may often respond to CPR if it is initiated soon after the lightning exposure.

ASSESSMENT

All children with burns, electrical injuries, or lightening strike injuries should be assessed and managed in the same manner as all trauma victims.

1. Scene survey
2. Airway, c–spine control, and initial LOC
3. Breathing
4. Circulation
5. Brief exam of abdomen, pelvis, and extremities
6. Critical transport decisions
7. Package and transport interventions
8. Secondary survey

Scene Survey

When approaching a burn victim, survey the scene to determine if there is a safe approach to the child. Also determine if any special equipment is required. The immediate priority in caring for the burn victim is to remove the child from the burning source. *The health care provider must be careful, however, not to become a victim also.* The child should be safely removed from the source of heat. This often will require the aid of fire personnel. Burned clothing and any constricting jewelry should be removed from the child. In addition, the wounds should be *briefly* irrigated with cool water so that the burns do not continue to act as a heat source and increase the underlying injury. Ice should never be directly applied to a burn injury.

In the case of electrical injuries, the child should be removed from any live electrical source. Here again, experienced rescue personnel and the power company may be required for a safe extrication. If there are chemicals involved, health care personnel should approach the child only when it is determined that there is no risk to the rescuer. The burns should be thoroughly irrigated after any dry chemicals have been brushed from the skin.

Airway and C-spine

As with any other trauma victim, if there is concern about the mechanism of injury, the mechanism of injury is unknown, or the patient has an altered mental status, manual c–spine control should be taken as soon as possible. The priorities in assessment and management should be the ABCs of any pediatric burn victim.

The rescuer must keep in mind special considerations that arise in assessing the ABCs of a pediatric burn victim. While assessing the child's airway, remember that children rescued from an enclosed area are at particularly high risk for airway compromise.

Clues suggesting possible airway injury include severe facial burns, singed eyebrows and nares, oral or pharyngeal burns, sooty sputum, hoarseness, or stridor. Close attention should be focused on the status of the airway in these children. Remember that because of the smaller cross–sectional area of a child's trachea, only a small amount of swelling can significantly obstruct the airway. Remember that any child with an obstructed airway should be repositioned immediately, the airway should be suctioned, and bag–valve–mask ventilations should be initiated where appropriate. If the child is not breathing, bag–valve–mask ventilations should be initiated immediately.

Breathing

The child's efforts at breathing should be assessed next. Determine the depth and rate of respirations. Any sternal or intercostal retractions, wheezing, cough, grunting, stridor, drooling, or hoarseness are troublesome signs in a burned child. Hypoventilation, respiratory distress, and respiratory arrest are common in patients with burns complicated by inhalation injury. Respiratory arrest is also seen in patients exposed to high–voltage electrical injuries and lightning strikes. Pulmonary injuries may also be seen in children burned after an explosion.

All children should receive 100% oxygen. In addition to correcting the hypoxemia the child may have been experiencing, this will begin to decrease the patient's carbon monoxide level.

Circulation

Next, the circulatory status is addressed. The child's circulation is assessed by comparing pulses in the neck and wrist. As discussed in Chapter 6, consider the child's level of consciousness, skin color, and temperature in addition to the pulse rate and quality of the pulses. Shock is rare in the early stages after a burn. Generally, burn shock takes several hours to develop and is caused by a shifting of fluids from the vascular system into the the burned tissue. If it is determined that a child is in shock after a burn injury, possible sources include internal bleeding following falls or automobile collisions, spinal shock caused by high–voltage electrical injuries (more than 1000 V), and myocardial damage resulting from electrical current.

The absence of pulses indicates a child in cardiac arrest. If it is determined that the child has no detectable pulse, immediate CPR should be initiated. This can occur with severe inhalation injury, high–voltage electrical injuries, and lightning strikes. Once cardiac arrest is recognized, a monitor/defibrillator should be applied. Children with electrical injuries present in ventricular fibrillation; those injured by lightning develop asystole as the result of prolonged respiratory arrest. Standard ACLS protocols should be followed in this setting. *Remember that these are usually young, healthy patients who will respond to resuscitation efforts if the duration of the cardiac arrest has not been too long.* Survival after prolonged resuscitation has been reported.

Brief neurologic assessment. If the child has an *altered mental staus,* stabilize the ABCs as quickly as possible and package and transport. In children with an altered level of consciousness after an inhalational injury, high levels of both carbon monoxide and cyanide may be present. The presence of these substances cannot be determined in the prehospital setting. Treatment should be initiated prior to confirming the presence of these agents. Prehospital treatment of carbon monoxide includes 100% oxygen delivered by tight–fitting nonrebreather mask. This hastens elimination of carbon monoxide from the body.

Critical Transport Decisions

As discussed, the initial concern in pediatric burn victims is with the child's airway, breathing and circulation. If any signs of an unstable airway, obvious respiratory insufficiency, shock, or an altered mental status are present, package and transport the child as quickly as possible.

Package and Transport Interventions

Airway and c–spine. Monitor children carefully for such signs of upper airway obstruction as tachypnea, stridor, or drooling. Endotracheal intubation must be established early because airway problems can develop suddenly in a child with even a small degree of airway obstruction. Children with trouble handling their secretions, an altered mental status, or extensive facial and oral burns also should have their airways secured with an endotracheal tube. When possible, intubations should be performed en route to the hospital. Intubation should be performed in the usual manner, except that an endotracheal tube 0.5 mm to 1.0 mm smaller than would normally be inserted, based on the age of the child, should be used. Prolonged and difficult attempts at intubation should be avoided, however, to prevent further damage to the child's airway. Sedation may be preferred due to the possibility of laryngoscopy–induced obstruction.

Breathing. Monitor the child's respiratory status very carefully during transport. Give 100% oxygen and watch for signs of respiratory distress or failure.

Circulation. If the child presents with a thready, rapid pulse and signs of shock, seek causes other than burns. In addition to oxygen therapy, IV access is essential for all burn victims. Children with burns suffer massive fluid losses during the early hours after their burns. Ideally, two large–bore IV lines should be established in peripheral veins, preferably in areas uninvolved by burns. IV access should be established *during transport* and should not delay removing the patient from the scene of the burn injury.

In addition, prolonged attempts to establish access are not warranted and may be delayed until arrival at the hospital, particularly if transport times are less than 30 minutes.

Begin aggressive fluid resuscitation as discussed in Chapter 6 if the patient shows any evidence of shock. The initial bolus should be 20 mL/kg of either lactated Ringer's or normal saline.

Care of the burn itself requires little specific attention. Covering the child with a clean, dry sheet is appropriate. Any provider who handles the patient should wear both gloves and a mask to prevent contamination of the burn wounds by microorganisms. Antibiotic ointment should not be applied during the prehospital phase of care.

Thermoregulation. In addition to covering the burns, keep the child warm during evaluation and transport. Because of their large surface area and small muscle mass, young children do not conserve body heat efficiently. When they suffer burns, their ability to conserve body heat is compromised even further, and hypothermia can develop. Finally, although children with burns may complain of thirst, they should be given nothing by mouth.

Cardiac monitoring. Children in shock or those with high–voltage electrical injuries or lightning strikes should have continuous cardiac monitoring because of the high incidence of cardiac dysrhythmias.

Secondary Survey

Once a thorough assessment of the ABCs is conducted, a more complete secondary assessment is made. Again, the provider should attempt to identify any injuries that have complicated the burn injury. Head, chest, neck, lung, and abdominal injuries can be seen as the result of falls, collisions, explosions, and high–energy currents that complicate the burn injury.

BURN WOUND MANAGEMENT

Extent and depth of the burn must be assessed in the burned child.

Extent

In the adult, the extent of injury is determined using the "Rule of Nines," which assigns multiples of 9% to certain areas of the body to calculate the total body surface area of the burn wound (Figure 11.2). This simple rule is not accurate for children, however, because they have a proportionately larger head and proportionately smaller lower extremities than adults.

As a result, the Lund Browder diagram is more useful in determining the body surface area of the burn in children (Table 11.1).

Another helpful rule to know is that the child's palm is equal to approximately 1% of the body surface area. For smaller burns, the extent of injury is estimated by determining how many of the palms would be equal to the area of the burn.

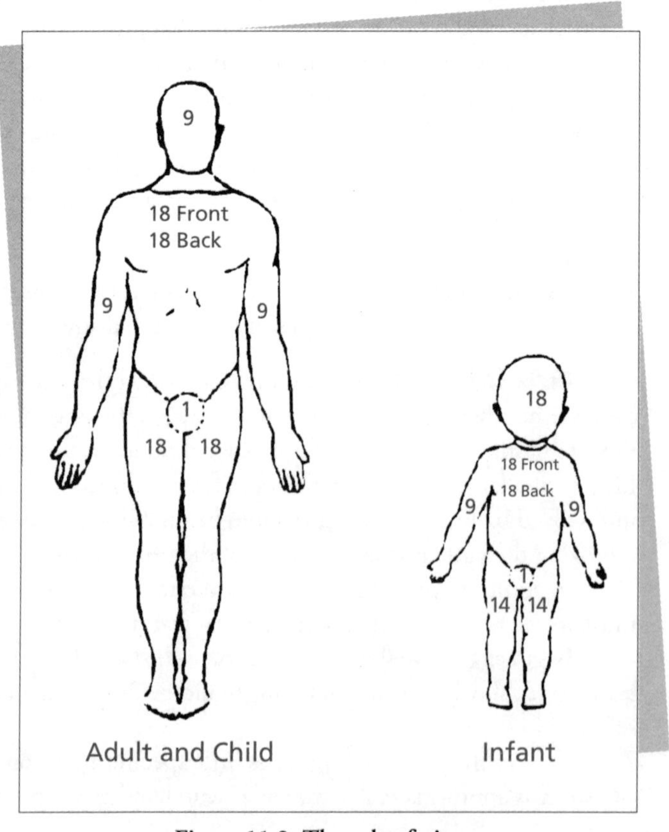

Figure 11.2. The rule of nines.

Area	Age (Years)					%	%	%
	0-1	1-4	5-9	10-15	Adults	2°	3°	Total
Head	19	17	13	10	7			
Neck	2	2	2	2	2			
Ant. Trunk	13	17	13	13	13			
Post. Trunk	13	13	13	13	13			
R. Buttock	2 1/2	2 1/2	2 1/2	2 1/2	2 1/2			
L. Buttock	2 1/2	2 1/2	2 1/2	2 1/2	2 1/2			
Genitalia	1	1	1	1	1			
R.U. Arm	4	4	4	4	4			
L.U. Arm	4	4	4	4	4			
R.L. Arm	3	3	3	3	3			
L.L. Arm	3	3	3	3	3			
R. Hand	2 1/2	2 1/2	2 1/2	2 1/2	2 1/2			
L. Hand	2 1/2	2 1/2	2 1/2	2 1/2	2 1/2			
R. Thigh	5 1/2	6 1/2	8 1/2	8 1/2	9 1/2			
L. Thigh	5 1/2	6 1/2	8 1/2	8 1/2	9 1/2			
R. Leg	5	5	5 1/2	6	7			
L. Leg	5	5	5 1/2	6	7			
R. Foot	3 1/2	3 1/2	3 1/2	3 1/2	3 1/2			
L. Foot	3 1/2	3 1/2	3 1/2	3 1/2	3 1/2			
				Total				

Weight ______________

Height ______________

Table 11.1. Lund Browder diagram.

Depth

The depth of the injury is determined by inspection of the burn wound. Burns are characterized as superficial partial–thickness (first–degree), deep partial–thickness (second–degree), and full–thickness (third–degree) depending on the amount of injury to the dermis and epidermis (Table 11.2).

Superficial partial–thickness burns extend through the epidermis and occasionally into the upper layers of the dermis. These burns appear red and dry and are painful. Because the lower layers of the epidermis tend to be spared by the burn, these wounds tend to heal on their own in ten to 14 days. Deep partial–thickness burns extend deep into the dermis. They appear red and wet, often have blistering of the skin, and are painful. These wounds often require some degree of skin grafting to heal completely.

Full–thickness burns extend through the dermis. These burns are white or charred in appearance due to the coagulation of skin and blood vessels (eschar). Because the nerve endings are destroyed, these burns are usually painless. Thesy do not heal without skin grafting and can be particularly troublesome when they extend around the chest or an extremity. Swelling below the eschar in a limb can create a tourniquet–like effect, leading to neurovascular compromise. Circumferential full–thickness chest burns can cause respiratory compromise. Because children have thinner skin than adults, they tend to experience deeper burns when exposed to the same amount of heat.

	Superficial partial thickness (1st degree)	**Deep partial thickness (2nd degree)**	**Full thickness (3rd degree)**
Layer	epidermis	epidermis dermis	all layers
Color	bright red	pale red	white or charred
Blisters	none	large	dry
Pain	moderate	severe	none
Healing	3 to 5 days	1 to 3 weeks	never
Scarring	none	moderate	severe

Table 11.2. Types of burns.

Fluid Resuscitation

Aggressive fluid therapy is important in the early stages of a burn. In thermal burns, lactated Ringer's can be given at an initial rate estimated by multiplying 0.25 by the child's weight (kg) times the percent body burn. As an example, the initial infusion rate in a 10–kg child suffering a 20% body burn is 50 mL/hr (0.25 x 10 kg x 20%). This formula is not appropriate for victims of electrical burns because the underlying tissue damage cannot be accurately determined by the surface burn. Fluid infusion of 20 times the child's body weight can be used. In the example above, an initial infusion of 200 mL/hr would be initiated for an electrical burn.

Pharmacologic Therapy

As discussed earlier, children who are victims of smoke inhalation may have been exposed to certain toxins such as carbon monoxide and cyanide. The initial therapy for carbon monoxide consists of supplying the patient with 100% oxygen to hasten elimination from the body.

Cyanide poisoning is treated safely using sodium thiosulfate solution. Sodium thiosulfate comes as a 50–mL vial of a 25% solution. Thirty mL (8 g) is given to a child less than 12 years old, and 50 mL (12.5 g) is given for a child 12 years or older.

Transport Considerations

The vast majority of pediatric burn victims should be transported to the closest available emergency department for initial stabilization. Only those children who have significant traumatic injuries associated with their burns need to be transported directly to a specialty care center. Children with extensive deep partial–thickness and full–thickness burns; burns involving the hands, feet, genitals, or face; burns complicated by inhalation injury; high–voltage electrical injury; or lightning injury will ultimately be transferred to a pediatric burn center.

Burn Prevention

Many factors place a child at unnecessary risk for burn injury. These include single–parent families, overcrowding, inadequate child supervision, and failure to promptly notify the local fire department.

Smoke Detectors

Smoke detectors are among the most effective interventions available for reducing smoke inhalation and burn injury. When used correctly, detectors are thought to reduce the potential for serious injury by up to 66%. Ongoing education needs to be provided regarding the effectiveness of smoke and fire detectors and their use.

Education

Children should be instructed about the dangers of electrical injury. Parents should minimize a child's access to electrical plugs and wires. Any area that has electrical wires should be forbidden to children. Climbing trees and flying kites in these areas are particularly dangerous.

During lightning, children should be taught to seek shelter inside and to avoid high places and open areas. They should also avoid metal fences.

Points to Remember

1. The first priority in a pediatric burn victim is to separate the child from the source of the burn. Remove all burned clothing, and take off any constrictive jewelry. Cool the burn injury with a small amount of cool fluid. Brush off any solid chemicals and use generous irrigation for all chemical injuries. *Do not become a victim!*
2. As with other trauma victims, first assess the child's airway, breathing, and circulation. Significant injuries are often associated with burn injuries. Do not overlook these injuries because of the dramatic appearance of the burns.
3. Be aggressive in managing the child's airway if signs of respiratory distress are present. Airway problems may suddenly worsen in children with upper–airway injury.
4. Shock in the early stages of a burn is not caused by the burn injury. Look for other sources of shock.
5. Fluid resuscitation should be initiated early in the pediatric burn victim. The rate of infusion is based on the child's weight and extent of burns. Children with high–voltage electrical injuries should receive more aggressive fluid resuscitation than suggested by the surface burns.

Suggested Reading

1. Dimick AR: Burns and electrical injuries, in Tintinalli JE, Krome RL, Ruiz E (eds): *Emergency Medicine: A Comprehensive Study Guide.* New York, McGraw–Hill, Inc., 1992.
2. Sumchai AP: Thermal burns, in Harwood–Nuss A, Linden C, Luten RC, et al (eds): *The Clinical Practice of Emergency Medicine.* Philadelphia, JB Lippincott, 1991.
3. Linden CH: Smoke inhalation, in Harwood–Nuss A, Linden C, Luten RC, et al (eds): *The Clinical Practice of Emergency Medicine.* Philadelphia, JB Lippincott, 1991.
4. Chabot DR, Gross PL: Lightning injuries, in Harwood–Nuss A, Linden C, Luten RC, et al (eds): *The Clinical Practice of Emergency Medicine.* Philadelphia, JB Lippincott, 1991.
5. Phillips LG, Robson MC: Emergency care of burn injuries, in Callaham ML (ed): *Current Practice of Emergency Medicine.* Philadelphia, BC Decker, 1991.
6. Jones J, McMullen MJ, Dougherty J: Toxic smoke inhalation: Cyanide poisoning in fire victims. *Am J Emerg Med* 1987;5:318.

Pediatric Drowning and Near-drowning

Richard N. Nelson, MD, FACEP
Nancy Asp, RN, EMT

Introduction

Drowning is a major preventable cause of death in the world today. Of the 140,000 drowning deaths worldwide each year, approximately 8,000 occur in the United States. Drowning is the third leading cause of accidental deaths in children of all ages.

Drowning is defined as death by suffocation from submersion in a liquid medium, usually water. Near–drowning is survival, at least temporarily, after submersion. While the submersion incident may occur as a result of readily explainable factors such as exhaustion or inability to swim, a precipitating event or associated condition is often present. This event or condition, if properly recognized, may have a profound effect on how the child is managed in both the prehospital and the emergency department settings.

ANATOMY/PATHOPHYSIOLOGY

Drownings can be divided into four categories: wet drowning, dry drowning, post–immersion syndrome, and immersion syndrome.

Wet Drowning

Wet drowning occurs when water is aspirated into the lungs as a result of the victim losing protective airway reflexes or because of inability to suppress respirations.

Freshwater aspiration constitutes the majority of drownings. Because fresh water is less concentrated than plasma, water aspirated into the lungs is quickly absorbed into the circulation via simple osmotic forces, resulting in hypervolemia. Thus, a child pulled from the water after aspirating fresh water may have little water left in the lungs by the time resuscitation is started. Of far more importance is the damage that freshwater aspiration causes to the lung tissue. Water disrupts surfactant activity, washing this important surface–active material from the alveolar membranes. As a result, alveolar surface tension is increased and lung compliance is decreased, leading to poor ventilation and oxygenation. Later, alveolar capillary membrane leakage occurs and causes pulmonary edema and further hypoxia.

Salt water is three to four times more concentrated than plasma. Thus, when salt water is aspirated into the lungs, fluid from the circulation is actually drawn into the lungs through the alveolar capillary membranes, resulting in hypovolemia and pulmonary edema.

Children who have aspirated salt water may have large amounts of water still in the lungs at the time of initial resuscitation. Surfactant in the alveolar capillary membranes is similarly affected with salt water aspiration, and severe hypoxemia is common.

Polluted water aspiration compounds the problems previously discussed. Chemical irritation of the alveolar membranes produces an inflammatory response in addition to direct damage to the alveoli and surfactant. In addition, children who have aspirated polluted water are more prone to later infections.

Dry Drowning

Approximately 10% of drownings occur without aspiration. Apparently, laryngospasm prevents water from entering the lungs, resulting in death by airway occlusion or asphyxiation rather than by aspiration. Theoretically, these patients have a better chance of successful resuscitation because the lungs are spared direct damage. In the prehospital setting, wet drowning cannot be differentiated from dry drowning.

Post–Immersion Syndrome

Whereas most submersion victims have immediate respiratory compromise, some patients are stable shortly after rescue only to develop respiratory distress later. This respiratory distress after an initial recovery period is referred to as post–immersion syndrome. Also called "secondary drowning," this syndrome usually occurs within 12 hours, but can appear up to 72 hours after submersion. Post–immersion syndrome is probably a form of acute respiratory distress syndrome (ARDS) caused by the pulmonary injury incurred during aspiration. Because it is impossible to predict who will develop post–immersion syndrome, it is essential that all patients who have experienced a significant submersion event be transported to the hospital and observed for at least 24 hours.

Immersion Syndrome

Sudden death occurring as a result of contact with water, usually cold, is known as immersion syndrome. This poorly defined syndrome is probably the result of vagal–induced cardiac arrest or bradycardia with loss of consciousness. Alcohol ingestion is considered a predisposing factor.

ASSESSMENT

All patients involved in a drowning incident should be considered multiple–trauma patients. Follow the standard pediatric BTLS approach.

1. Scene survey
2. Airway, c–spine control, and initial LOC
3. Breathing
4. Circulation
5. Brief exam of abdomen, pelvis, and extremities
6. Critical transport decisions
7. Package and transport interventions
8. Secondary survey

Scene Survey

Is the scene safe? If the child is still in the water, are there any dangers in getting the child out? Rescuing children who have fallen through ice is particularly treacherous, and each year many would–be rescuers become victims themselves after being submerged in ice water.

Another potential hazard is malfunctioning electrical equipment (lights, heaters) in home swimming pools. Electricity transmitted through the water may not only have caused the victim to drown, but may be a potential hazard to the rescuer.

Airway and C–spine

Cervical spinal cord injury with paralysis or a head injury with loss of consciousness may prevent even the expert swimmer from staying above the water. Common causes of aquatic head and neck injuries include head–first dives into shallow water, surfing and water skiing accidents, and auto and boating accidents.

Always pay close attention to the c–spine. If there has been a history of trauma, if there is evidence of trauma (cuts or bruising on the head, face, or neck), or if no history is available, assume there is a c–spine injury and take manual control of the c–spine.

Mouth–to–mouth ventilation may be started on the apneic submersion victim while still in the water. Once the child is out of the water, aggressive resuscitation efforts begin. If the patient is apneic or having inadequate respirations, open the airway using the modified jaw thrust maneuver and attempt to ventilate with a bag–valve–mask. If forced ventilation is difficult or impossible, suspect an airway obstruction.

Never perform a blind finger sweep on a child.[1] Use the maneuvers suggested for the removal of a foreign body in an infant or child. Remove the object only if it is visualized, and ventilate the child between attempts at foreign body removal. Have suction ready, as these maneuvers may precipitate reflux of water from the lungs or stomach resulting in aspiration.

Breathing

If the child is being ventilated, always use 100% oxygen. Always assume hypoxic brain injury and hyperventilate the child. Do not waste valuable time trying to "drain" water from the lungs. In freshwater submersion, most of the aspirated water will probably have been absorbed through the lungs into the circulation. In a salt water submersion, there may be water in the lungs; however, time is better spent on airway control and ventilation than on trying to "drain" the lungs.

The child who is awake and able to protect his own airway should be placed on a 100% nonrebreather mask. Carefully monitor these children for signs of respiratory failure.

Circulation

If a pulse is not present, begin CPR immediately. If a pulse is present, determine the rate and check for the capillary refill. Stop all active sources of bleeding.

Brief neurologic assessment. Although the lungs are affected first, the brain is most susceptible to permanent damage from cerebral hypoxia. All resuscitation efforts should be directed at getting oxygen to the brain. Children may appear entirely normal after submersion or may appear dead with no movement and no pupillary responses. Between these two extremes are confusion, combativeness, obtundation, decorticate posturing, and decerebrate posturing. Beware of the fact that a head injury, alcohol or drugs, seizures, or hypoglycemia can result in an altered mental status and may complicate drownings.

Critical Transport Decisions

Rapidly package and transport any child with an unstable airway, respiratory insufficiency, shock, or an altered mental status. Attempt to resuscitate any child who has been submerged for an hour or less, particularly if the water is cold. Children who have fallen through ice may become hypothermic very quickly, and this hypothermia may offer some protection against anoxic brain injury. There have been a number of case reports of children who are victims of cold water drownings surviving even after prolonged submersion times. Children in cardiac arrest following cold water submersion require transport to a hospital capable of instituting advanced rapid rewarming techniques, including cardiopulmonary bypass.

Package and Transport Interventions

Airway and c-spine. The most important actions in resuscitating critical submersion victims are control of the airway and ventilation with 100% oxygen. Any child who is apneic, unconscious, or inadequately ventilating should undergo endotracheal intubation. Such intubation should be performed orally by the most experienced person present, while maintaining c–spine immobilization. If the patient's airway is open, keep him on 100% oxygen during transport. An unresponsive child with a Glasgow Coma Scale score of less than 8 should be intubated to protect the airway and provide for better oxygenation of the brain.

Apply appropriate cervical immobilization as soon as feasible. During the log roll of the child onto the backboard, be careful to avoid movement of the c–spine and assess the back of the child.

Breathing. If the child is intubated, make sure the endotracheal tube is correctly positioned and there are equal breath sounds bilaterally. If the child is not intubated, carefully monitor the respiratory status during transport. If the child is hypothermic, warmed, humidified oxygen may be used. If a pulse oximeter is available, use it to maintain the oxygen saturation above 95%, preferably 100%.

Circulation. Attach the child to a cardiac monitor. Cardiac arrhythmias are common in submersion victims because of the combination of hypoxia, acidosis, and hypothermia. Cardiac arrhythmias are treated according to the ACLS guidelines, with one important exception. If the child is severely hypothermic [less than 86° F (30°C)], the heart may not respond to cardiac medications. Therefore, in the presence of severe hypothermia, only one course of ACLS drugs should be given prior to the time the child is warmed to 92°F(33.9°C). IV access should be obtained en route to the hospital. IV fluids should be run at a keep–open rate unless the child shows signs of shock. Fluid boluses should be kept to 10 mL/kg to avoid aggravating head and pulmonary injuries from excessive fluids.

While en route to the hospital, remove all wet articles of clothing and attempt to keep the child warm.

Thermoregulation. Hypothermia is a common finding in submersion victims, particularly children, whose body surface (heat exchange) area to body mass (heat generating) ratio is greater than that of adults. Because the body loses heat much faster when immersed in water than air of comparable temperature, hypothermia develops quickly. Immersion hypothermia occurs in both summer and winter.

In general, hypothermia should not be treated in the field. However, it is possible to prevent further heat loss and worsening hypothermia in a child by removing wet clothes, drying the child, and wrapping him in blankets.

Use warmed IV fluids and warmed, humidified oxygen, if available on the vehicle. Severe hypothermia [less than 86°F (30°C)] must be managed aggressively, because some children who have fallen through ice and been submerged for prolonged periods have survived neurologically intact. These children should be rapidly packaged and transported to a hospital capable of providing cardiopulmonary bypass.

Secondary Survey

While en route to the hospital, perform a secondary survey if time allows. Start with the head and finish with the extremities. Pay special attention to the neurologic examination. Note the level of consciousness, pupillary reaction, and motor and sensory response.

Transport the child quickly to the nearest appropriate facility, calling ahead to allow the emergency department time to prepare for the patient's arrival.

SPECIAL CONSIDERATIONS

Certain events, such as c–spine injury, head injury, use of alcohol or drugs, seizures, hypoglycemia, and child abuse, may initiate a drowning or near–drowning episode. Seizures, even while the child is in shallow water, may result in aspiration and subsequent drowning. Children with a seizure disorder have a fourfold increase in drowning risk. Hypoglycemia with loss of consciousness while in the water may lead to a drowning event, particularly in diabetic children. Although diabetic children are usually carefully controlled, extra exercise or poor eating, both of which may occur during the summer, can lead to hypoglycemia. Child abuse should be suspected when submersion events occur under questionable circumstances, such as in bathtubs, buckets, or toilets.

The prehospital provider is in a unique position to gather important historical information and observe the accident scene. Careful observation and documentation will provide important information to the emergency physician and appropriate authorities.

PROGNOSIS

Warm–Water Drownings

Victims with submersion times of less than 5 minutes who develop return of spontaneous circulation within 10 minutes of ACLS resuscitation will likely have good outcomes. Factors thought to adversely affect outcome include prolonged submersion, delay in the initiation of CPR, severe acidosis, asystole on arrival at a medical facility, fixed and dilated pupils, and unresponsiveness (Glasgow Coma Scale score less than 5). *Children who arrive at the emergency department with CPR in progress have a dismal outcome.*

Cold–Water Drownings

Falls through ice or submersion in water less than 40°F(4.4°C) offer the best chance for full neurologic recovery. Adults tend to struggle, panic, and drown when they are submerged. Children are more likely to be caught unaware and offer no struggle, and this may result in their brains being protected as their body temperature drops rapidly.

Hypothermia may result from one of two situations. The first is a "true" cold–water drowning in which the child falls through ice. Because severe hypothermia greatly reduces cerebral oxygen requirements, the brain may be able to withstand anoxia for a longer period. These children have been reported to survive neurologically intact even after being under the water for an hour. Cold–water drownings require aggressive resuscitation and transport to a pediatric center.

The second situation that may result in severe hypothermia is brain death. As the brain dies, the ability to control body temperature is lost and the patient becomes progressively cold. This diagnosis should never be made in the field, and all these patients should be transported to a skilled pediatric center.

PREVENTION

Drowning now outranks motor vehicle collisions or pedestrian trauma as the single leading cause of injury and death in children less than 5 years old. Recent legislation and public information campaigns targeted to the use of child seats and restraints is largely responsible for this disparity. National attention now needs to focus on prevention of drowning because nearly all drowning deaths are preventable.

Most drowning deaths occur in private pools, either at the child's own home or at a neighbor's. It has long been believed that parental supervision is the key to drowning prevention. Even so, as history has proven, it takes only a momentary lapse in supervision to result in catastrophe for a child. Other protective mechanisms must be present to "save" the child during lapses of parental supervision.

Pool Enclosures, Covers, and Alarms

Complete pool fencing has emerged as a promising prevention strategy. More stringent laws governing total pool closure are needed in most states. This means installing a fence no less than 4 feet high on all sides of a pool. A house cannot be considered the fourth side of the pool enclosure because children would then have direct access to the pool. The fence must also have a self–closing, self–latching gate. At the time of this writing, only 15% of in–ground pools in the United States had complete pool fencing.

Pool covers are designed only to retain heat in pools and hot tubs and to keep debris out. Young children may climb onto the covers, slip beneath them, and drown. More rigid pool covers have been advocated, but because their application can be cumbersome, few are in use in the United States today.

Pool alarm systems have recently been evaluated by the Consumer Product Safety Commission. No satisfactory system exists, and further study is needed.

Public Information Campaigns

Because prompt resuscitation is vital to survival, pool owners should be mandated to learn CPR. All too often, bystanders pull children from the water and wait for emergency medical service personnel to arrive and initiate CPR.

Health care providers can teach parents to empty their buckets after chores, to never allow children to bathe alone without adult supervision, and to enroll their children in swimming classes at an early age.

Points to Remember

1. Childhood drowning is largely preventable with common sense and education.
2. Early, aggressive CPR, rapid airway management, and transport to a pediatric center offer the best hope for survival from drowning.
3. Children submerged in cold water [<40°F (4.4°C)] have a better chance for survival than those submerged in warm water.
4. States should strongly consider mandating fencing around pools.

Bibliography

1. Beyda DH: Prehospital care of the child with a submersion incident. *Crit Care Nursing Clin North Am* 1990;3:281–285.
2. Modell JH: Drowning–current concepts. *N Engl J Med* 1993;328:253–256.
3. Orlowski JP: *Submersion Injury,* vol 9. Elk Grove Village, Illinois, American Academy of Pediatrics, 1989, p 1–10.
4. Quan L: Drowning issues in resuscitation. *Ann Emerg Med* 1993;22:366–368.
5. Wintemute GJ: Drowning in early childhood. *Pediatr Ann* 1992;21:417–421.

Pediatric Trauma Arrest

Steve Shaner, EMT–P
William Cotton, MD

Introduction

The pediatric trauma arrest is defined as cardiorespiratory arrest occurring as a direct result of physical trauma to one or more body systems.

According to the National Pediatric Trauma Registry, one half to two thirds of all pediatric trauma deaths occur before the patient reaches the hospital. Trauma arrest in the adult population has a near 99% mortality rate. While there is less information on trauma arrest in children, pediatric trauma arrest may have a lower mortality rate due to the child's natural response mechanism. A look at 584 traumatized children who received CPR in the prehospital setting showed that 450 of the patients died. However, 134 survived to discharge from the hospital. While morbidity data were not available, these figures may suggest that, with proper intervention, pediatric trauma arrest has a slightly better outcome than in adults.

As in medical arrests, the primary cause of trauma arrest is usually due to airway or respiratory compromise. If hypoxia is ignored in the trauma patient, it may lead to respiratory arrest. The airway must be maintained and oxygen delivered to prevent hypoxemia.

Circulatory compromise may also lead to arrest. A prolonged insult to the vascular system may cause the vital organs to die as a result of hypoperfusion. Early recognition and prompt intervention may control the body's response to shock and prohibit needless morbidity or mortality.

A rapid, well–organized assessment is the key to recognizing possible causes of trauma arrest. Interventions can then be used to stop or reverse a potentially fatal situation.

CAUSES OF TRAUMA ARREST

Airway obstruction
Hypoxia
Tension pneumothorax
Hemorrhagic shock
C–spine fracture
Aortic transection
Pericardial tamponade
Electrical shock

ASSESSMENT

The assessment of the child in trauma arrest is the same as in any other situation and should be performed in the following order:

1. Scene survey
2. Airway, c–spine control, and initial LOC
3. Breathing
4. Circulation
5. Brief exam of abdomen, pelvis, and extremities
6. Critical transport decisions
7. Package and transport interventions
8. Secondary survey

Scene Survey

The mechanism of injury may provide valuable information regarding the cause of the arrest. Carefully investigate the scene for clues that may suggest how the actual injury occurred.

Airway and C–spine

An uncorrected airway obstruction may lead to a respiratory arrest followed by a cardiorespiratory arrest. An obstructing tongue or a foreign body obstruction can usually be relieved by basic airway maneuvers. Suctioning blood and mucus from the oropharynx may also be necessary to maintain a patent airway. An airway obstruction must be cleared before the assessment is continued. Manual c–spine control must be maintained due to the possibility of injury.

Breathing

Hypoxia, regardless of the cause, must always be considered when dealing with the trauma arrest. One cause of arrest, while not common, is tension pneumothorax (Figure 13.1), a life–threatening situation that can be corrected in the prehospital setting. Rapid needle decompression will usually be life–saving. Administration of 100% oxygen and airway management are also essential.

C–spine fractures may also lead to respiratory failure and even arrest. Airway management with c–spine control must be used.

Circulation

Hemorrhagic shock may also lead to arrest. All acute external hemorrhage must be controlled. Signs of abdominal injury could point to massive intra-abdominal bleeding. CPR should be initiated if the pulse rate or blood flow is not adequate to perfuse the brain.

Pericardial tamponade, although a rare condition, may also be treated with proper recognition and rapid transport. Cardiac arrest caused by electrical shock may often be treated successfully. Ventricular fibrillation induced by electrical shock may be treated using pediatric ACLS protocols. Defibrillation, as well as consideration of associated trauma, may be life–saving.

Critical Transport Decisions

The trauma arrest is always a situation in which the rescuer must make a time–versus–benefit decision. The decision to transport to the closest appropriate facility by ground or by air may be a difficult one. It may be helpful to contact your regional pediatric trauma center for more information. Trauma arrest is always a rapid package and transport situation.

Package and Transport Interventions

The approach to management of the trauma arrest must be aimed at treating the cause of arrest. All standard packaging interventions must be established before transport.

Airway/breathing. Initially, airway compromise and hypoxemia should be treated. Basic airway management, suctioning, and bag–valve–mask ventilations must be initiated. If basic airway management is not effective and the patient needs more definitive airway management, endotracheal intubation should be performed. If basic airway maintenance is effective, intubation may be accomplished in transport. If tension pneumothorax is suspected, trained providers should perform needle chest decompression. All victims of arrest should be ventilated at a rate of eight to ten breaths per minute more than their normal respiratory rate.

Circulation. Circulatory compromise must also be addressed. If no pulse exists, perform CPR. If cardiac tamponade or massive hemorrhage is suspected, the patient should be packaged and transported as soon as possible. Temporizing therapy such as pneumatic antishock garment inflation and IV/intraosseous fluid resuscitation should be initiated en route to the hospital. A rapid survey of the abdomen, pelvis, and lower extremities should be completed before application of a pneumatic antishock garment.

Pediatric ALS protocols should be followed in cases of cardiac arrest that do not respond to aggressive airway management and fluid resuscitation. The use of defibrillation and one round of cardiac medications may be appropriate if airway management and fluid resuscitation have been unsuccessful.

Secondary Survey

In a trauma arrest situation, there may not be sufficient time to perform a secondary survey. If the cause of the arrest cannot be determined, the secondary examination may reveal subtle clues as to the etiology of the arrest.

Points to Remember

1. Early recognition and intervention are the key to reversal of trauma cardiorespiratory arrest.
2. Appropriate care may increase the chances for survival of those victims who would otherwise die from their injuries.

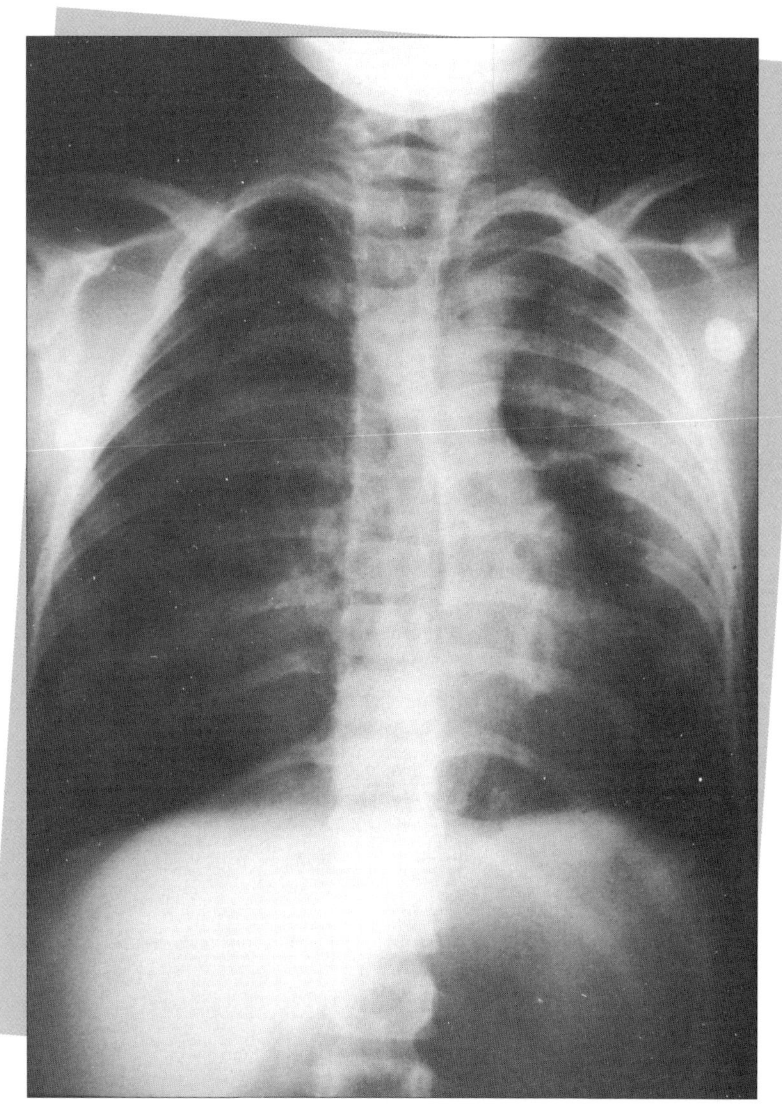

Figure 13.1. Tension pneumothorax.

Child Abuse

Jeanette Foster, MSW

Introduction

Child abuse (the nonaccidental injury of a child) is no longer a problem that emergency medical personnel occasionally encounter in the field. It is a national emergency. As these encounters increase in frequency and as people generally become more sophisticated about how to manipulate abuse injuries and histories to avoid detection, it becomes vital for prehospital care providers to be aware of indicators of abuse, recognize high–risk families, obtain pertinent information, and convey this critical information to the appropriate authorities.

Prehospital care providers at the scene have a number of advantages as gatherers of information. They are privy to initial explanations for an injury, often before a consensus by members has been reached. They are able to notice the environment in which the alleged accident occurred, and they are in the company of assorted family and friends, most of whom will not come to the emergency department. These advantages place prehospital care providers in a unique position to detect or suspect nonaccidental injury to a child.

Initially, it is important to listen to all stories given for the injury. Do not assume that the family was "so upset they couldn't think straight." Although that may also be true to some extent, *different* explanations for an injury should be documented. The greater the discrepancy between the stories, the more concerned the provider should be. For example, you are called to the home of a family in which the child has just sustained a head injury. The mother says that she, the child, and the father were playing and the child struck his head. She leaves the room to get her coat, and the father walks in and says that *only* he and the child were playing and the child fell down the steps. It would be prudent to begin to recognize the discrepancies between these two stories as a potential problem. It is not uncommon for a husband or wife to cover for each other, or for family members or friends.

In addition to noting the discrepancies between stories and documenting them, the provider should assess the likelihood of the explanations. As a parent describes a scalding tub burn, notice the tub, its height, the height of the faucets, type and location of faucets, etc. Is the child's developmental ability consistent with the story? A 9–month–old is not generally considered able to turn on a faucet, close the drain (allowing water to pool), and climb into the tub. Take advantage of your ability to scope out the territory of the alleged accident and make some notes.

This is a good time to remember that child abuse can happen in *any* family. Some families may have more chronic patterns of abuse; some may generally function well but with acute stressors experience a breakdown in normal coping abilities and abuse the child. Remember to pay attention in homes that seem "safe" or "nice," because on those occasions prehospital providers are most vulnerable to attributing inconsistencies to stress, "believing" far–out stories, etc.

Children are hurt and killed in all kinds of homes. However, there are some indicators associated with high–risk households, including neglect (filth; lack of heat, food, clothes, and supervision) and the presence of drugs, alcohol, or weapons. Observations of these conditions should be documented factually. The presence of large groups of observers at a scene also increases the likelihood that a prehospital care provider will be told something that a well–meaning family member communicated to the hospital. Pay attention to these stories and keep them in the back of your mind.

Ideally, private, individual histories should be obtained, but rarely do emergency medical personnel have this luxury. In general, the history is obtained from those present while the injuries are being treated. The ride to the emergency department can be a good time to ask a parent or the child (if the child feels safe) about the history of the injury.

Red flags that may suggest nonaccidental injury are inconsistent history and injury; changing histories to find the "right" explanation; witnesses who report abuse; a child who demonstrates excessive fear or withdrawal from a particular person(s); other indicators of acute stress, including wreckage (after a domestic violence episode), financial problems, marital problems, member with a chronic medical problem, drugs/alcohol, isolation; a child who reports being abused.

Characteristic marks that may indicate possible physical abuse include unexplained injuries accompanied by marks with the appearance of such man–made objects as belts, belt buckles, cords, and spatulas; cigarette burns; pinch marks; adult–size bite marks; immersion straight–line burns; rope burns; and burns in the shape of heated forks, spoons, irons, etc, on unlikely body surfaces (back of the hand, back, leg, or face). Unexplained mouth or dental injuries, fractures (especially in infants), or unexplained abdominal or head trauma, should raise the suspicion of abuse. Head injuries and abdominal injuries are the first and second most common causes of death, respectively, as a result of abuse in infants and toddlers.

CARE AND SAFETY ISSUES

In situations where abuse is suspected, chances are the family members present will show some signs of anxiety as they attempt to avoid detection. There is tremendous family pressure to not disclose information and to minimize the damage done. The decision to transport the child can be difficult.

While some children will automatically be taken to the emergency department for assessment and treatment of their injuries, others may not require a medical evaluation. When abuse is suspected, consider transporting the patient. The trip to the emergency department may be the only means of assessing the history, injury, and the family's reaction to it. *The child's safety is of paramount importance!* If resistance to transporting the child is met at the scene, stress to the family the need for emergency department assessment of the child. In situations of suspected abuse, some families may refuse treatment or transportation of the child. Follow local procedures in such instances, including an immediate report to law enforcement of concerns and suspicions. Should law enforcement personnel agree with the assessment of emergency medical personnel, they can remove the child and allow transport to the emergency department for evaluation. Again, it is imperative in suspected abuse cases to minimize additional trauma to the child. One of the easiest ways to manage this is to calmly assess the situation and transport the child whenever possible to the emergency department for assessment and case management. *Do not confront family members with discrepancies at the scene; just listen and remember.* If the child is in a dangerous situation and parents are demanding that you leave, contact your supervisors or law enforcement for assistance.

EMERGENCY PERSONNEL CONSIDERATIONS

Families will be anxious, afraid, and often defensive following the nonaccidental injury of a child. It is expected that emergency personnel will experience many emotions and thoughts regarding a family who abuses, or allows the abuse of, one of their children. It is perfectly normal to feel a wide range of emotions, including anger, toward the family. Allow yourself to have opinions and feelings but remain objective in your tasks of information gathering, assessment, and treatment. Not only will your calmness prevent further emotional escalation in the family and further trauma to the child, but members may actually *tell you something.* A person feeling guilty may share some of the guilt with a nonthreatening prehospital care provider. Gather information calmly and relay it to the emergency department.

FAMILY MEMBERS' EMOTIONS

Although there are a number of different presenting characteristics for family members of an abused child, the primary motivating emotion is generally fear. The consequences of being discovered may include jail, disruption of family, income loss, jeopardized marriages, further domestic violence, and rejection by family and friends. For many, there is also the fear of not being discovered and knowing that the abuse will continue and worsen. When people are afraid, their normal coping patterns work less efficiently. They are more apt to become violent, fight, flee, or lose control. The primary task of prehospital care providers is to remain calm and in control. The quickest way to diffuse an individual who is on the verge of losing control is to be calm and stable.

Other family reactions may include increased domestic tension, arguing, pacing, drinking, drug use, or flight. Should any of these or other reactions interfere in the treatment of the child or become a personal threat, contact supervisors and/or law enforcement agencies.

A way to defuse family members' reactions is to assure them of your concern for the family. "I am concerned about the child and you, but I can only tend to the child right now." This will place them in a position of being supportive of you. Allow families to ask questions. Give them concrete answers. People under stress hear and remember approximately 10% percent of what they are told, *so keep it simple.*

Continually reassure family members that you are caring for their child and that the child will be transported to the emergency department for a comprehensive evaluation.

EMERGENCY DEPARTMENT

On arrival in the emergency department, it is essential that all the information gathered is shared with the appropriate people. If the child is transported to an emergency department in which a social worker is present, the information should be conveyed to that individual. If a social worker is not available, give the information to the charge nurse and/or attending physician(s).

If the child is not transported to the emergency department, but there are suspicions about the incident, report your concerns to the appropriate law enforcement and protective service agencies. Prehospital providers do not have to prove anything they suspect; they only need to *suspect* it to report it.

Points to Remember

Many obstacles, such as concerns about retaliation, paperwork, or going to court, and conflicts with law or protective services personnel, may deter individuals from reporting child abuse. The only real loser in unreported child abuse is the *child* who is reabused and, perhaps, killed.

1. Any suspicious event or incident should be reported to the proper authorities for investigation.
2. All information gathered at the scene should be given to the emergency department staff.
3. Do not confront the family at the scene.
4. Report all suspected abuse.

Suggested Reading

1. Hodge D III, Ludwig S: "Child homicide:" Emergency department recognition. *Pediatr Emerg Care* 1985;1:1.
2. Kingman R: Child abuse and neglect: Critical first steps in response to a national emergency. *Am J Dis Child* 1991;145.
3. America's children: How are they doing? Fact sheet. American Humane Association, Children's Division, May 1993.

Pediatric Trauma Triage and Major Incident Management

Jim Augustine, MD, FACEP

Introduction

Management of major pediatric trauma incidents requires a different approach from that of adults. The mechanisms of pediatric injury are typically accidental, not intentional, and may involve a strong emotional response from responsible adults. It also may evoke a strong emotional response from rescuers. A well–organized incident management system will minimize the emotional component and allow a confident evaluation and treatment plan to be carried out.

Dealing with any major EMS incident, especially one involving multiple seriously injured children, requires a uniform approach to facilitate both the medical and psychological evaluation of all of the involved children. The uniform assessment, interventions, packaging and transport methods emphasized in this course should be utilized to optimize efficiency and care.

ESTABLISHING PRIORITIES FOR INCIDENT MANAGEMENT

Major incidents involving children with serious or critical trauma, or incidents involving multiple children will influence triage priorities. Often times prehospital providers will prioritize children for treatment and transportation over adults. This is a natural response to guide the highest level of care towards the pediatric class of victims that may be perceived as more salvageable. This response is predictable and should be considered by Incident Command and other sector officers during the operation. If an adult and child have similar injuries, for example, a closed head injury with airway compromise, the pediatric victim will be prioritized for transport before the adult patient.

When an incident involves an entire family unit, pediatric priorities will influence decisions regarding institution and mode of transport. A sector officer involved in making transportation decisions must, if possible, keep a family unit together to facilitate information gathering and ultimately the medical care of the individual family members. Examples of incidents where this type of situation may occur include: multiple family members injured in an automobile or other vehicular accident, or carbon monoxide inhalation. *Whenever possible, if it does not overwhelm the receiving hospital, all family members should be taken to the same facility.* Family members may then provide support and medical information for each other. This can become complicated when there are separate pediatric and adult trauma facilities serving the area where the incident occurs. Decisions should be made based on the severity of the injuries and local protocols. If the family must be divided between institutions obtain as much information as possible prior to transport and the phone number of another relative that may be contacted to stay with the child.

If the parent refuses to be separated from the child, be calm, explain the options and that missed injuries can be devastating for a child. EMS personnel should not unnecessarily overload one facility in such a way that medical care for all the family members is compromised.

MANAGING PEDIATRIC MULTIPLE CASUALTY INCIDENTS

Incidents involving multiple pediatric patients are not uncommon. Several common scenarios include: school bus accidents, chemical exposures in schools, motor vehicle accidents where a large number of children are in the same automobile, or exposure to environmental poison. EMS personnel are challenged during these incidents to triage the victims with the most serious illness or injury from those who are upset, anxious, or perceiving a medical problem. These events can challenge the diagnostic skills of the emergency responder, but also challenges the patience of that provider. Episodes of mass hysteria may occur, where suddenly there are large numbers of victims requesting evaluation and transportation. Resources may not be available to provide immediate transportation for all those who feel they are ill or injured, or may compromise the care of those who have life–threatening injuries. In these circumstances, several incident management techniques are of use.

1. A member of the emergency response team should establish themselves as being in charge of the incident (Incident Command) and a triage leader should be designated. These individuals should establish themselves as the authority and direct all communications and proceedings.

2. Potential victims, or those complaining of an illness or injury, should be physically separated from those who are uninjured.
3. Those victims who are most seriously ill or injured must be transported away from the scene as rapidly as possible.
4. An emergency responder with good communication skills should be appointed to reassure the other members of the group and try to prevent any panic reactions or undue anxiety.
5. At an appropriate time, all individuals involved in the incident who wish to be evaluated should have a complete assessment performed and documentation completed. This ensures that each patient receives a comprehensive evaluation. Frequently the assessment is reassuring to those individuals involved in the incident and is an appropriate time to advise them to get follow–up for any psychological issues that may develop.
6. An authority recognized by the group, such as a school authority, team leader or school counselor may be valuable in reassuring the group and preventing undue anxiety.

Considering these pediatric differences, the management of multiple casualty incidents proceeds according to established management principles of triage, treatment and transportation.

Preplanning for an incident will establish resources that will be available when an incident occurs. Incident command may appoint an individual to gather all needed equipment, supplies, and personnel for the incident. These individuals must assess the need for resources and plan accordingly. When estimating what resources may be needed, try to over–estimate to insure that the needs of the rescuers are met.

Triage may be defined as doing the best for the most with the least effort, in the shortest amount of time. Triage is utilized in any accident involving more than one victim. Two rescuers should be assigned to do primary triage. Primary triage consists of checking the ABCs of each victim. If any insufficiency is noted in the ABCs or level of consciousness, the victim must be tagged as a "Priority I." If there are no obvious deficits in the ABCs but other obvious injuries exists, the victim should be tagged a "Priority II." Victims who are stable and ambulatory should be tagged as a "Priority III."

After primary triage is completed, secondary triage and extrication must be completed. Secondary triage includes treatment of immediate life threatening injuries – Priority II patients may also have to be upgraded to areas where they can be more definitively treated. Priority III should be directed to an area where a more detailed exam can be performed.

Once proper triage has been performed, other trauma scoring methods may be used to assist with direction of seriously injured patients to pediatric tertiary care centers. Unnecessary deaths and debilitating injury can be reduced if proper triage is performed on every multi–casualty incident.

Treatment and transportation of pediatric trauma patients must proceed in a timely manner. Consideration should be made to the climate, distance from hospital and victims' condition. In general, prehospital providers should err on the side of rapid packaging and transportation.

Early airway stabilization is mandatory, but establishing IV lines, wound care, and application of MAST are less important and can be applied during transportation or at the hospital.

As much information as possible should be provided to the receiving facility, particularly if multiple victims are involved, this will allow the hospital to mobilize the appropriate equipment and personnel. As mentioned, an attempt at keeping the family together should be considered if care will not be compromised.

Field management of pediatric patients is summarized in **Figure 1.**

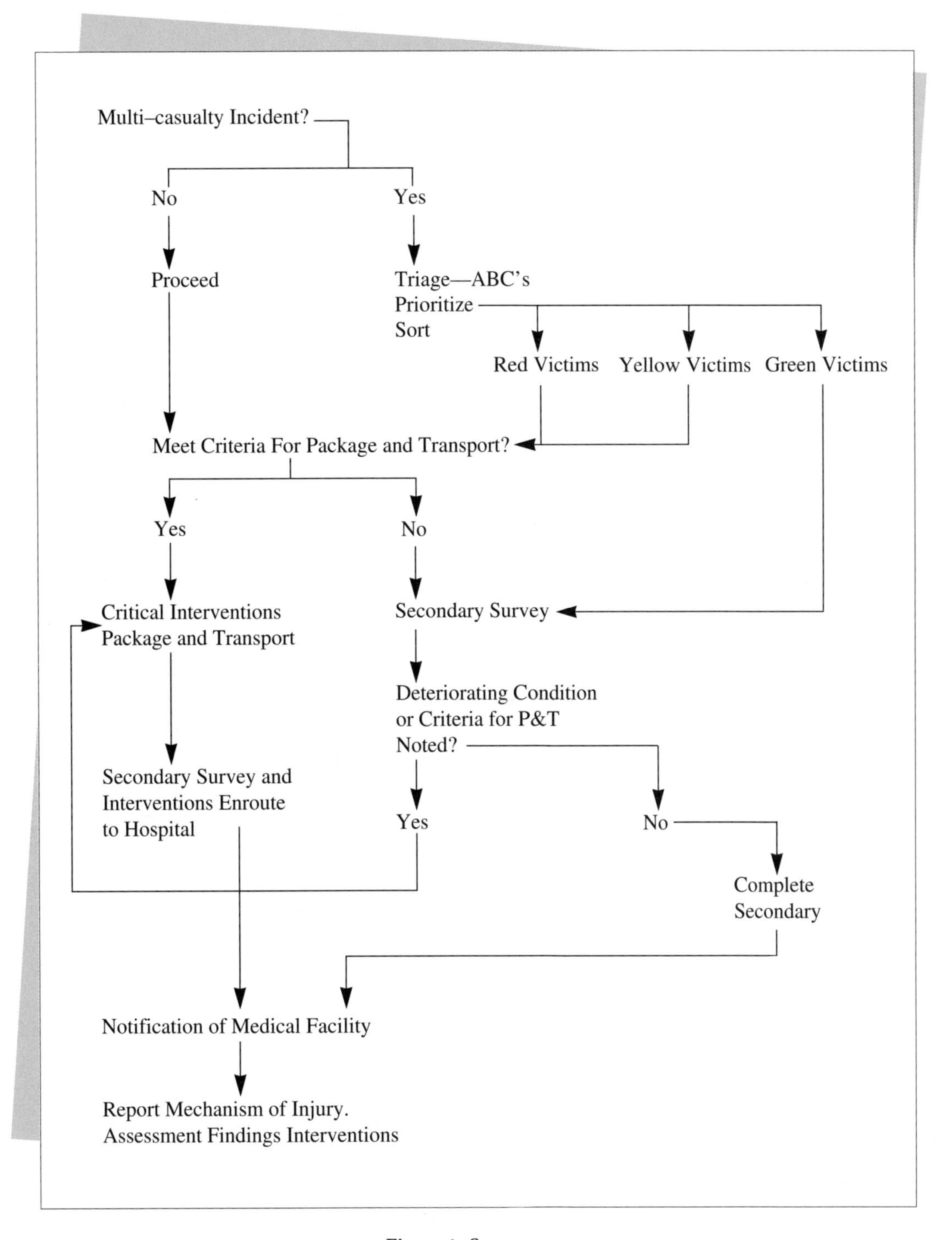

Figure 1. Scene survey

PEDIATRIC CONSENT & MAJOR INCIDENT MANAGEMENT

The issue of consent for pediatric patients in major incidents may be raised. The consent issue in these circumstances is usually less complicated than in routine day–to–day operations. In major incidents, there is an anticipated higher level of anxiety and concern for the pediatric patients. The usual rule of "implied consent" for evaluation and treatment may be evoked. The EMT is acting on behalf of society to evaluate and provide appropriate treatment for pediatric patients who otherwise cannot provide their own legal consent unless emancipated. The responder is therefore acting in a legally responsible manner when a pediatric patient assessment is performed. If the EMT feels that treatment is required immediately, there is no need for parental consent. An excellent example of this would be a major commercial airline crash where there are multiple victims of varying ages. A child found in the wreckage would be assumed to have significant injuries until proven otherwise. This child who is temporarily separated from the parents for whatever reason should be appropriately evaluated by the EMS responder. If that responder found any indication of illness or injury from the crash, the child would be immobilized and then transported without first attempting consent from any parents. Should the parents later be located, consent for treatment may be obtained retrospectively. Even if this type of consent could not be obtained, the EMT operated in a responsible fashion considering the potential mechanisms of injury and their primary concern for the physical well–being of the patient.

This "implied consent" does not force the EMT to provide transportation and treatment to all pediatric patients who are not accompanied by a parent or guardian. It is only permissive in allowing the EMT to perform appropriate functions that, in the best judgement of the EMT, are necessary for evaluation.

For example, a car full of seventeen year old students involved in a motor vehicle collision at a low rate of speed may generate an EMS response for evaluation. Considering the mechanisms of the accident, the EMS providers evaluate these students and find no evidence of any injury. Unless there is some indication of injury, no transportation or treatment will need to be performed on these patients. These patients cannot legally sign a release document for non–transportation but can be instructed and expected to understand about seeking further medical care should any symptoms of an injury develop.

EQUIPMENT CONSIDERATIONS

Multiple casualty incidents often result in a shortage of packaging and treatment equipment. When this occurs, pediatric specialized equipment may not be available for each child.

Children cannot be expanded to fit on or into adult size equipment and adult size equipment cannot be condensed in the field. Pediatric sized equipment must be used for the appropriate sized child whenever possible. A variety of manufacturers offer equipment especially designed for children. Child size airway equipment, cervical immobilization devices and spinal immobilization equipment is available. On occasions where sufficient equipment is not available, improvisational techniques may be employed, ensuring that the objectives of the interventions are met. The skill/intervention sections of this text will assist with learning to select the appropriate equipment.

PSYCHOLOGICAL EFFECTS

Major incidents involving pediatric patients can be expected to generate a higher degree of psychological stress among the response personnel than incidents involving adults. Critical incident stress debriefing teams should be utilized and made available for counseling. If this resource is not in the community, a counseling team from the regional pediatric trauma center may be available. Appropriate debriefing is very important for pediatric cases, and to prevent long term psychological trauma, home problems or unnecessary job anxiety related to future pediatric patients.

Points To Remember

To effectively manage major pediatric trauma incidents, the following steps are utilized:

1. Identify incident as a major or multiple casualty incident.
2. Establish incident command and appropriate sectors.
3. Call for needed medical and rescue resources.
4. Adequate and appropriate triage.
5. A rescue command in charge of extrication and medical person in charge of each victim.
6. Adequate preparation with appropriately trained personnel to do victim care and airway control.
7. Professional communication and interaction of incident command personnel is necessary. This should be facilitated through the use of the extrication table and agreement among the sector officers.
8. Appropriately timed hospital notification will enhance medical care and turnover of the patient to the hospital.
9. Debrief after the incident to learn, ask questions, minimize stress and learn for the next incident.

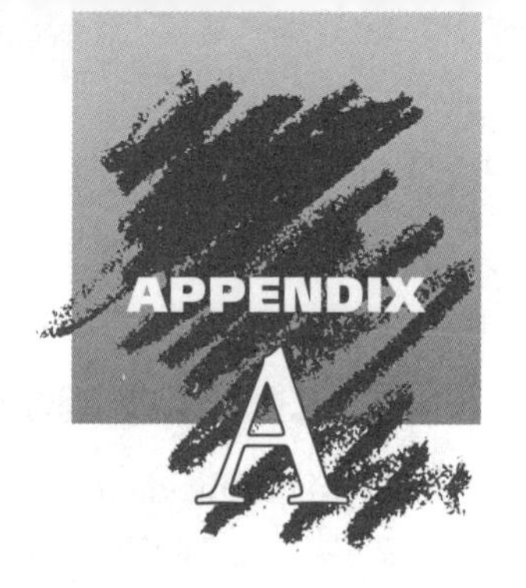

Death of a Child

Nancy Nelson, MSW

Introduction

There is perhaps no crisis more emotionally challenging and stressful for emergency medical personnel than the critical injury or death of a child. Not only are emergency personnel challenged by arduous medical tasks, they often are also confronted with overwhelming demands from parents and families, who are thrust into an unexpected and catastrophic event. The death of a child in our society is often regarded as the "ultimate tragedy." Children are not supposed to die, certainly not before their parents. The death of one's child is potentially the most profound and devastating experience of one's life. Although the nature and specific circumstances surrounding a child's death can be very different, parental reactions are overwhelmingly similar. Even where differences do occur, most can be considered acceptable and expectable within a wide continuum of reactions.

The following have been identified as three stages in the initial process of grief with which emergency personnel may need to deal: shock – the initial response, demonstrated by denial, numbness, internal conflict, and guilt; affective/emotional reaction – the internal experience or outward expression of anger, sadness, fear, or anxiety; and alpha mourning – the beginning process of mourning, which involves the perception, expression, and acknowledgement of catastrophic loss.

Through these initial stages, parents, family members, and close friends of critically injured and dying children may display the following behaviors: tearfulness, hysterical crying, flatness of affect, and labile behavior that vacillates between different and extreme displays of emotion; angry or hostile reactions that may appear to be directed toward emergency personnel; and feelings of guilt, hopelessness, and loss of control over oneself and the situation.

GRIEF REACTIONS

Certain somatic symptoms are often present in acutely grieving parents and can complicate the emergency medical personnel's role as care giver to the child. The parent who exhibits any of the following symptoms may require emergency medical evaluation as well as support: rapid, tense speech; shortness of breath, chest pain; tension headaches, muscle spasms, and nausea; loss of strength and faintness; restlessness and hyperactivity; hypertension; and confusion and impaired concentration.

Sudden death generates a different kind of grief, "a harsher variety" than in the case of death after a long illness. Accidental deaths and other kinds of sudden loss are more difficult because there is no opportunity to prepare for the loss. Intensified guilt and self blame are common feelings for parents whose children are injured in accidents that they feel they could or should have prevented.

When confronting these intense reactions in others, it is important to identify your own feelings. Care givers may identify with particular people or situations. For example, a 5–year–old child who dies may be particularly upsetting for care givers with children of the same age. The immediate reaction may be to distance oneself from the grieving family as the intensity of their emotion is overwhelming. Care givers may fear being blamed because they could not save the child, or they may fear not knowing the answers or what to say to the family. It is important to acknowledge your own feelings of powerlessness and helplessness.

Critical incident stress debriefing may be very beneficial for health care providers following a trauma that results in a death or intense emotions in the providers.

COMPASSIONATE FRIENDS

Compassionate Friends is a self–help organization offering support for bereaved parents and families. They have made several suggestions for how people can help when a child dies. The following suggestions have been adapted from their literature.

1. Don't try to find magic words that take away the pain; there aren't any. A hug, a touch, and a simple "I'm so sorry" offer real comfort and support. Be comfortable with silence.
2. Don't be afraid to cry. Sometimes tears express what words cannot.
3. Avoid saying things like "I know how you feel" unless you also have lost a child and have experienced the same depth of loss.
4. Don't try to find something positive in the child's death such as "at least you have other children" or "God must think you are very special to handle this." There are no words that make it all right that their child has died.
5. Avoid judgments of any kind. Saying "you should..." or "you shouldn't"... is not helpful.
6. Be patient. Remember that different people respond differently to pain. Some scream, others withdraw and are unable or unwilling to talk. Others strike out angrily.

7. Be willing to ask about the child. Even though you may have never known the child, many parents will cherish the opportunity to tell you through their tears how special their child was. This can also be helpful to you as you resolve your own feelings about the death.
8. If possible, give some special attention to surviving children who may be present. They are hurt, confused, and often ignored. Many older children will suppress their painful feelings to avoid adding to their parents' pain. Talk to them and acknowledge their loss.
9. Be aware that a child's death can raise serious questions about God's role and the parents' religious beliefs. Ask the family if they have a pastor or minister whom they would like you to contact. Do not presume others' religious beliefs are like your own.
10. Listen, listen, and listen!

There are some additional recommendations that Compassionate Friends makes for emergency medical personnel and first responders who are in the position of notifying parents of the sudden death of their child.

First, identifying information should never be released to the news media prior to family notification. A family member hearing of a child's death by TV or radio is catastrophic. Second, the family should never be notified of the death of their child by telephone. Ideally, at least two personnel should make the notification. One should be a provider of information, and the other should be available to observe the reaction of the family. This team should break the news in steps.

1. Confirm identify of family members.
2. Tell them there has been an emergency.
3. Tell them that the situation was so serious that a death occurred. Promptly give information about the incident, i.e., car accident, fall, etc.
4. Use the child's name if possible and provide specific, clear information tactfully and honestly.

After notification, family members should not be left alone. Offer to contact neighbors, friends, clergy, and others who can be present to provide support and assistance.

In situations in which a dying child is transported to the hospital, the family is often waiting for what seems like a very long time for information. Although the clinical responsibilities may seem overwhelming, make some contact with the child's family.

If the child is not doing well, prepare the family gently for bad news. Repeated visits with updated information, even if it is bad, can reduce the trauma to the family. Make sure appropriate hospital staff and social workers and/or the chaplain are aware of the family's situation. These individuals may provide the family with support and convey their important needs and wishes to the care givers. If possible, after the child has expired and the family is departing, give the family a name and phone number to contact with their unanswered questions.[4]

Remember, the death of a child is potentially one of life's cruelest and most devastating blows. Responders have the challenge to provide care not only to the child, but to the child's loved ones. Your patience, honesty, and the capacity to listen to the most painful and overwhelming feelings the family is experiencing enable parents to begin to grieve and allow their emotional wounds to begin the long process of healing.

Points to Remember

1. The death of a child is an emotionally challenging experience for emergency medical service personnel.
2. Acute grief reactions include tearfulness, hysterical crying, a flat affect, anger, hostility, and extreme displays of emotion.
3. Your patience and capacity to listen to the most painful and overwhelming feelings enables parents to begin the long process of grieving and healing.

Bibliography

1. Holland L, Rogich LE: Dealing with grief in the emergency room. *Health and Social Work* 1980;5:12–17.
2. Knapp RJ: *Beyond Endurance. When a Child Dies.* New York, Schocken Books, 1986, p 77.
3. How can I help when a child dies? The Compassionate Friends, Inc., 1987.
4. For first responders dealing with the sudden death of a child. The Compassionate Friends, Inc., 1988.

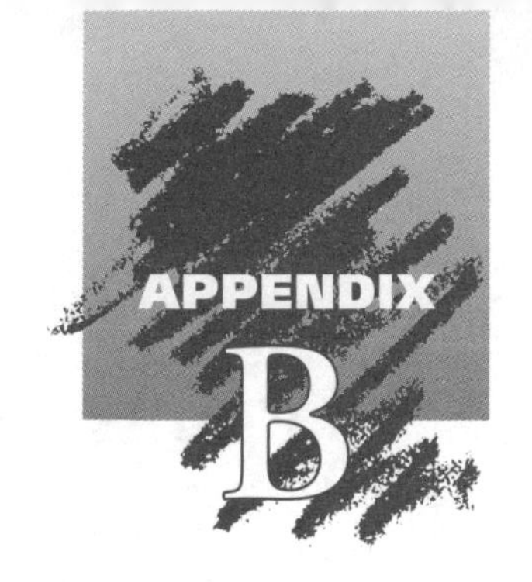

Trauma Scoring

Kathy Haley, BSN, RN
Bonnie Beaver, MD, FACS, FAAP

Introduction

Triage can be defined as "to pick, sort, or choose." To standardize the care giver's approach, a variety of triage scoring methods have been developed. In addition to these, there are also several assessment indexes/scoring methods that quantify morbidity and mortality for the injured patient. However, regardless of which method is used, most provide data to determine the following: triage of adult or pediatric victims to the right care facility, evaluation and monitoring of prehospital and hospital trauma care, research and clinical decisions, and epidemiologic trends/patterns.

Initially, using a scoring method may be time–consuming and actually may just confirm the frequently described "sixth sense" used by some emergency medical services personnel. In most cases, however, scores may be useful in providing direction to getting the right injured victim (triage) to the right place (definitive trauma center) during the right amount of time (mode of transport). Transport should never be delayed because of a lack of or difficulty in deriving a trauma score.

THE PEDIATRIC TRAUMA SCORE

Although controversy exists regarding whether a separate scoring method is needed for children, the Pediatric Trauma Score (PTS) is the only method designed for children. Developed by Tepas et al, the PTS is a combination anatomic–physiologic score.[1] The score is useful as a triage tool, a predictor of severity of injury, and a checklist that can quickly identify life– threatening or potentially life–threatening injuries. In addition to correlating well with the Injury Severity Score for recommendations for transfer to a Level I trauma center, it has been useful in predicting those patients in need of critical care resources.[2]

ASSESSMENT CRITERIA FOR THE PEDIATRIC TRAUMA SCORE

The PTS is determined by evaluation of six components and assignment of a severity (–1, +1, +2) level (Table B.1). The PTS ranges from a +12 (indicated minimal or absence of injury) to a –6 (indicating a fatal injury).

Severity	**+2**	**+1**	**-1**
Weight (used because of body surface to volume ratio factors that affect physiologic reserve)	> 44 lb (>20 kg)	22-44 lb (10-20 kg)	22 lb (< 10 kg)
Airway	Normal—A child whose airway is within normal limits and requires no supportive measures	Maintainable—A child whose airway is partially obstructed and who requires simple measure for protection (head positioning, oral airway, oxygen delivery by mask)	Unmaintainable—A child whose airway requires more definitive management (invasive procedure, intubation)
Blood pressure-systolic	> 90 mm Hg	50-90 mm Hg	< 50 mm Hg
(In the absence of blood pressure cuffs, palpated pulses may be used.)	Palpation of pulse at wrist (peripheral pulses)	Palpation of pulse in groin or neck, but not at wrist (central pulse only)	Absence of palpable pulses
Level of consciousness	The child who has had no loss of consciousness and is fully awake	Any degree of obtundation or history of loss of consciousness	Nonresponsive
Fracture	No evidence of fracture	Single closed fracture	Child with multiple fractures or an open fracture
Skin	No evidence of any trauma to the skin	Abrasion or minor injury to the skin	Penetrating injury, regardless of location, or a major avulsion or laceration

Table B.1. Pediatric Trauma Score.
(Source: Tepas JJ, et al. The pediatric Trauma Score as a Predictor of injury severity in the injured child. *J Pediatr Surgery* 1987; 22(1):14–18)

Once completed, all the numbers are added, providing a PTS score. A prehospital score of 8 or less indicates a critically injured child who should be transported to a trauma center.

PTS Example:

Scenario: You arrive at the scene after a 4–year–old child (weighing 18 kg) has been struck by a car. Assessment findings include a patent airway, respiratory rate of 38, capillary refill of 3 seconds, and rapid pulses palpable at the wrist. The child is alert and responds appropriately to questions. Assessment of the extremities reveals a 4–cm abrasion and deformity of the left thigh (you suspect a fracture). Using this information, calculate a PTS (Table B.2).

PTS Criteria	Actual Score	Rationale
Weight	+1	18 Kg
Airway	+1	Requires oxygen by mask
Blood pressure or pulse	+2	Palpable at wrist
Level of consciousness	+2	No history of loss of consciousness
Fracture	+1	Possible fracture femur (closed)
Skin	+1	Abrasion on the thigh
Total	8	Requires transport to trauma center

Table B.2. PTS calculation.

Points to Remember

1. Transport should *never* be delayed because of a lack of or difficulty in deriving a trauma score.
2. The PTS is the only method designed for children.
3. A prehospital PTS of 8 or less indicates a critically injured child who should be transported to a trauma center.

Bibliography

1. Tepas JJ, et al: Pediatric trauma score as a predictor of injury severity in the injured child. *J Pediatr Surg* 1987;22:14–18.
2. Aprahamian C, et al: Pediatric trauma score: Predictor of hospital resource use. *Arch Surg* 1990;125:1128–1131.

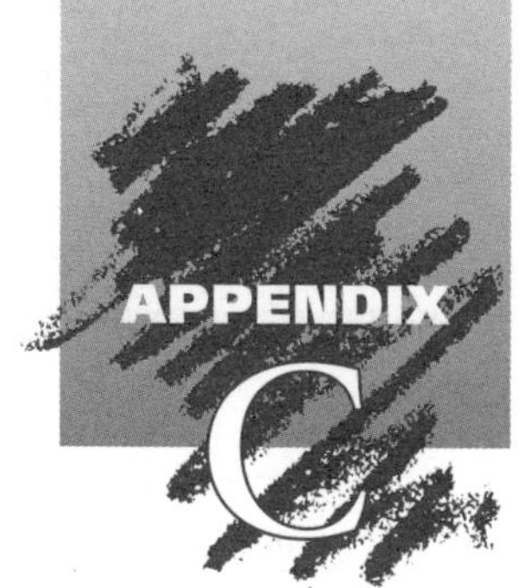

Use of Specialized Pediatric Care Centers

Howard A. Werman, MD, FACEP

Introduction

The vast majority of injured children may be appropriately managed at local medical facilities following a traumatic injury. On occasion, it is necessary to transfer a child to a pediatric trauma center or pediatric burn center for more specialized care than is available locally. The decision to transfer the child is often made after assessment and stabilization at the local emergency facility in consultation with the pediatric center. There are, however, instances in which direct transfer of the child from the scene of an injury to the pediatric trauma center or pediatric burn center is warranted.

DECISION PROCESS

The decision to transfer a child directly to a specialized care facility is based on two very important principles: speed and specialization. Children with significant multisystem trauma have a better outcome when those injuries are rapidly stabilized and repaired. The "golden hour" of trauma care applies in children as well! The child's outcome depends not only on the speed at which he is delivered to the health care facility but also the ability of that facility to provide resources that meet the child's needs. Pediatric trauma centers and pediatric burn centers have been established to provide that level of expertise to the injured child.

The decision to transfer a child directly to a specialized care center is one that requires a great deal of preplanning and should be approached with careful deliberation. Local facilities must often be bypassed during the transfer, raising important medicolegal questions. In addition, care in the specialized facilities can be quite costly. Finally, by removing the child from the "home" environment, important emotional and psychological support systems may be lost to the child.

Prehospital care providers should work with the medical directors to establish written policies to deal with injured children. Knowledge of area resources, including the capabilities of the local medical facilities, pediatric trauma center, and pediatric burn center, and the available methods of transport should be considered. The decision to transfer an injured child to a specialized facility should be made by the most medically experienced person at the scene.

Ideally, the decision should be made in consultation with on–line medical direction. In cases where this is not possible, written guidelines should be established by the emergency medical service medical director (see below).

GUIDELINES FOR DIRECT TRANSFER FROM AN INJURY SCENE

The American College of Surgeons and the National Association of EMS Physicians have established guidelines for direct transfer of the injured child from an injury scene. The guidelines detail anatomic, physiologic, and injury mechanisms that are associated with a high likelihood of significant underlying injury following trauma. The guidelines are summarized in Figure C.1.

Physiologic Criteria

Glasgow Coma Score ≤ 12
Pediatric Trauma Score ≤ 8
Patient who requires intubation
Shock secondary to trauma as evidenced by tachycardia, delayed capillary refill, and hypotension
Respiratory distress

Anatomic Criteria

Penetrating injury to head, neck, torso, or groin
Crushing injury to chest, abdomen, or head
C–spine injury
Abdominal trauma with significant tenderness
Two or more proximal long–bone fractures
Pelvic fractures
Limb paralysis
Amputation proximal to ankle or wrist

Mechanism of Injury

Ejection from automobile
Pedestrian struck by vehicle traveling more than 10 mph
Death of another occupant in the vehicle
Severe vehicle damage requiring extrication
Falls of more than 10 feet
Rollover motor vehicle accident
Automobile speed of more than 40 mph

Figure C.1. Transfer guidelines.

The guidelines suggested above provide direction in identifying pediatric patients who are at "high risk" for a significant injury. Clinical judgment must be used in every case. Some children who meet these criteria do not have evidence of any significant injury. On the other hand, other children with seemingly little trauma show evidence of severe injury.

Special mention must be made concerning the care of pediatric burn victims. As a rule, these children can be transported to the local emergency facility for stabilization and early treatment.

Even children who will ultimately end up in a pediatric burn center do not need to be transported directly from the scene to the specialized facility. The only exception to this statement is the child who has sustained major traumatic injuries as a consequence of the burn. Traumatic injuries may result from explosions, violent muscular contractions, and falls. These children should be transported as rapidly as possible to either a pediatric burn center or pediatric trauma center, depending on local protocol.

APPROPRIATE MODE OF TRANSPORT

Part of the decision process in transferring a child directly to a pediatric specialty center from the site of injury involves the selection of an appropriate method of transport. Two primary options are available for scene response: ground vehicles and helicopter. Selection of the appropriate mode of transport is based on the distance (and time) to the specialty center, local resources, weather conditions, and skills of the transporting agency. As with the decision to transfer, direct consultation with on–line medical direction or written protocols should be established to provide guidance in determining the appropriate transport mode.

Transport by ground ambulance is preferred when the time and distance to the pediatric trauma center or pediatric burn center are short. In general, ground ambulance should be used for transport distances of less than 15 miles or transport times of less than 30 minutes. Ground ambulance offers several advantages over helicopter transport. Ground transport is more cost–effective than air transport and is not generally affected by weather conditions. There is an orderly transfer of medical responsibility from the ground ambulance crew to the receiving physician when ground transport is used. In addition, there are fewer space constraints in a ground ambulance.

Helicopter transport is used for distances of between 15 and 100 miles or when transport times exceed 30 minutes. Despite their limitations, helicopters are useful in situations in which speed and the special skills of the crew are a consideration for patient care. Helicopters should also be considered when transport of the patient will occupy a community's local emergency medical services resources.

Airplane or fixed–wing transport is generally not used for direct scene transfer of children, except in the most rural environment. Airplanes are useful if the distance is in excess of 100 miles or the weather conditions do not allow helicopter transfer. In these settings, the patient should be transported to the local emergency facility for initial treatment and stabilization while awaiting transport.

Points to Remember

1. Most children can be treated at the local emergency facility following a traumatic injury.
2. Guidelines should be established for the direct transfer of significantly injured children from the accident scene.
3. The decision to transfer a child from the scene should be made by the person with the most medical experience on the scene in consultation with on–line medical direction.
4. The mode of transport is determined by the time and distance to the pediatric specialty center as well as weather conditions and local resources.

Bibliography

1. Air Medical Services Committee: Air medical dispatch: Guidelines for scene response. *J Disaster Prehosp Med* 1992;7:75–78.
2. Committee on Trauma: Prehospital triage criteria, in *Advanced Trauma Life Support Course for Physicians.* Chicago, American College of Surgeons. 1993.
3. American Academy of Pediatrics Committee on: Guidelines for air and ground transportation of pediatric patients. *Pediatrics* 1986;78:943–950.

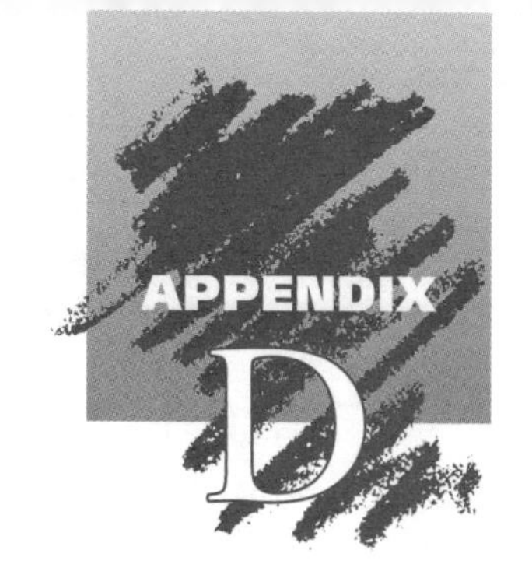

Pediatric Pre-existing Conditions

Katherine Shaner, RN, CEN

Introduction

As medical care has expanded and technology has improved, many children who might otherwise have required extensive management in a health care facility may be at home with their families. Premature infants who were 26 weeks gestation at the time of delivery may go home with their parents to a local community. In addition, many children have pre–existing medical disorders or are dependent on certain apparatuses. Prehospital providers and community hospitals must understand the specific needs and concerns of these children. If these children are involved in a traumatic incident, devastating injuries may result if their special needs are not included in their trauma care.

APNEA

Apnea is defined as any episode in which respiratory air flow ceases. The cause of this cessation may be central, obstructive, or mixed.[1] Central apnea is usually the result of central nervous system immaturity; as a result, the child "forgets" to breathe. Obstructive apnea is usually the result of a mechanical problem that makes the child unable to take a breath (i.e., in younger infants with poor head control, apnea may occur when the head falls into the chest).

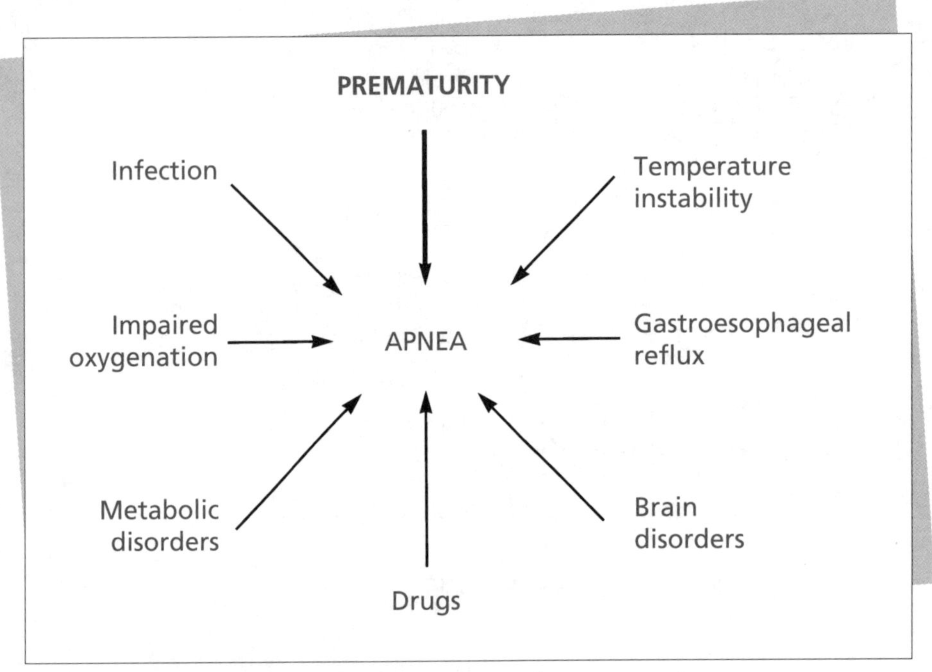

Figure D.1. Causes of apnea.

By definition, apnea in infancy refers to any unexplained episode in which breathing ceases for 20 seconds or more, or is associated with cyanosis, pallor, bradycardia, or limpness.[1]

There are many "causes" of apnea to be considered. They range from chalasia (relaxation of the muscle at the bottom of the esophagus allowing the child to vomit and inhibit respirations), to seizures, shock, hypothermia, sepsis, and trauma. A history of apnea is very significant to health care providers and should be taken as an indication of a possible serious illness.

Important questions to ask regarding these children are:

Was this a full–term infant, or was the baby premature?

How premature was the baby?

Did the baby need a "breathing tube" in the hospital?

How long did the apneic period last?

Did the baby change color?

Did the baby need stimulation to breathe again, or did he start on his own?

How many times has this happened?

These children need constant airway monitoring during transport. Take care in transporting a "sleeping comfortably" infant for apnea because this condition occurs primarily at rest. Frequent assessments of respirations, pulses, and skin color are needed. Pulse oximetry can be a very valuable tool for monitoring these children. When children have apneic spells, they usually desaturate (their oxygen saturation drops). If a child has an apneic episode during transport, stimulate the child, monitor the airway carefully, and intubate if necessary. Report any of these episodes to emergency department personnel. Apnea is usually a disease of the first three months of infancy. Children who had apneic episodes as an infant usually are not at risk for problems as they get older and can be treated as a normal trauma patient.

BRONCHOPULMONARY DYSPLASIA

Bronchopulmonary dysplasia (BPD) is a chronic lung disease occurring in premature infants who have survived neonatal respiratory failure.[2] These children have notoriously poor lung compliance, tachypnea and retractions at rest, and are barrel chested. The severity of the disease determines the amount of home therapy the child will receive. These children most often will be on home oxygen therapy and may receive home ventilatory assistance (Figure D.2).

Half of the children diagnosed with BPD will require hospitalization in the first two years after discharge from the nursery.[2] These children have a difficult time handling respiratory infections, and respiratory synticial virus can be particularly devastating.

Respiratory synticial virus is very common in the winter months and will severely exacerbate wheezing and respiratory distress. Other factors that may cause breathing difficulties for these children are smoking and environmental pollutants. Children who are on oxygen at home are at particularly high risk for developing respiratory difficulties.

Important questions to ask regarding these children are:

How premature was the infant?

How long was the child in the hospital?

How long was the child on the "breathing machine ?"

How much oxygen is the child on at home?

Does the child need mechanical assistance to breathe sometimes?

What medication does the child take?

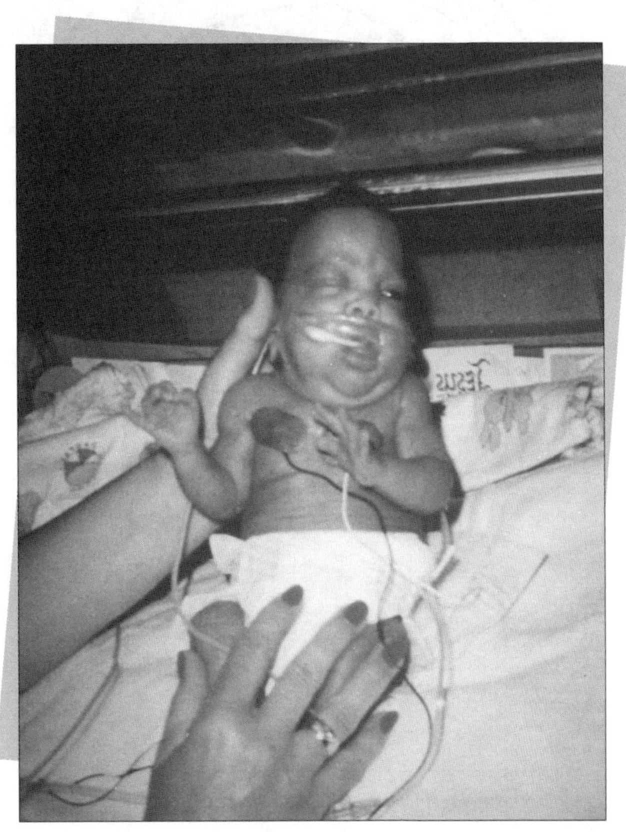

Figure D.2. Picture of child with BPD.

The parents of these children can be very valuable sources of information. Ask them to stay with the child and to assist while care is provided. Agitation makes these children much worse; so the calmer the child, the better the lungs will sound. If an aerosol is needed, allow the parents to hold it in front of the child. If the child requires spinal immobilization, keep the parents as close by as possible to reassure the child. These children may wheeze with stress and require an aerosol.

Airway patency is crucial during a BPD exacerbation. The care giver should be very aware of such signs of impending respiratory failure as increased respiratory effort, decreased aeration of the lungs, and increased fatigue from working too hard to breathe. Monitor these children carefully; most children in respiratory distress will be agitated. A "sleeping" infant or an infant with head bobbing who is in respiratory distress is an ominous sign. These signs do not mean a child is going to sleep; they mean respiratory arrest is imminent.

If a child with BPD is involved in an accident, carefully monitor the oxygenation and ventilation. Recognize that if this child requires intubation, he may need a smaller size endotracheal tube because of previous airway manipulations. The child may also be difficult to ventilate because of previous lung disease.

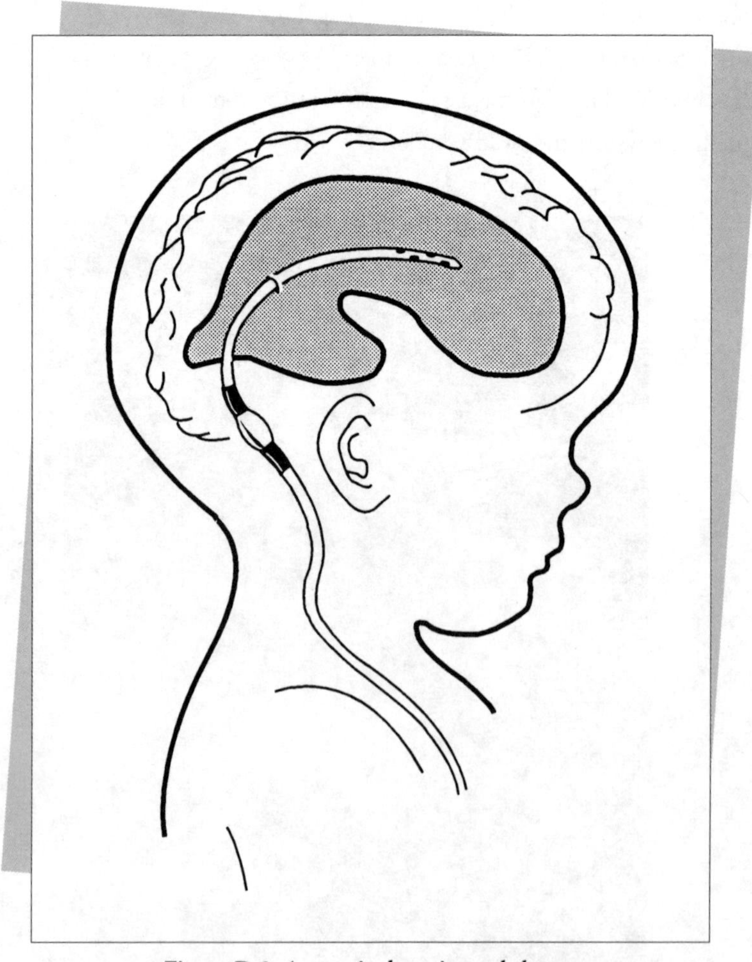

Figure D.3. A ventriculoperitoneal shunt.

SHUNTS

Ventriculoperitoneal shunts are placed in children to relieve hydrocephalus. Hydrocephalus is defined as a dilation of the cerebral ventricles, most often occurring secondary to obstruction of the cerebrospinal pathways and accompanied by an accumulation of cerebrospinal fluid within the skull.[3]

The ventriculoperitoneal shunt travels from the lateral ventricle through the skull to the subcutaneous tissue. It runs posteriorly to the ear and then continues subcutaneously to the abdominal cavity, where the cerebrospinal fluid drains into the peritoneal cavity (Figure D.3). If the shunt functions properly, the fluid is absorbed by the peritoneum.[4]

Important questions to ask regarding these children are:

On which side of the head is the shunt located, or does the child have bilateral shunts?

When was the shunt placed?

Has the shunt needed to be replaced?

Has the child been ill?

Is the child's activity level normal?

Does the child's shunt "pump" adequately, or does it seem sluggish?

Is the child acting the same as the last time the shunt didn't work? (Ask only for children with a history of shunt dysfunction).

When a child is dependent on a shunt for drainage of cerebrospinal fluid, a dysfunction may result in an accumulation of fluid within the ventricles, increasing intracranial pressure and creating devastating consequences for the child. The most common malfunction, by far, is obstruction of the shunt. In a significant number of children with shunts who sustain head trauma, even minor, the shunt will disconnect, with resultant dysfunction. All children with a shunt who sustain head trauma should be evaluated in an emergency department.

Children with nonfunctioning shunts will present with signs and symptoms of increased intracranial pressure (Figure D.4).

Signs and Symptoms of IIP
Headache
Irritability
Lethargy
Seizures
Bulging fontanelle

Figure D.4. Signs and symptoms of increased intracranial pressure.

These children may also complain of nausea, headache, and vomiting. Infants may have a characteristic "neuro cry" that resembles a kitten or cat yell; it is very high pitched and obviously abnormal. Seizure activity with shunt dysfunction is also a possibility.

Children with shunt dysfunctions should be monitored very closely for any signs of increasing intracranial pressure.

They need aggressive ventilation and airway management to assist in combating a rising carbon dioxide level and hypoxemia, which may lead to an increase in intracranial pressure. Seizure precautions also should be taken with these children.

If the child has any symptoms that the shunt is not working properly, or if the family believes the shunt is not working, the child should be monitored closely and transferrred immediately to an appropriate facility. *Shunt dysfunctions can be life–threatening and should be taken very seriously!*

TRACHEOSTOMIES

A tracheostomy is the insertion of an endotracheal tube to bypass marked narrowing of the larynx by structural anomalies, spasms, or inflammation of the trachea.[5] This procedure is used for long–term management of infants and children with noncorrectable airway obstruction or trauma of the airway.

Important questions to ask regarding these children are:

Why was the tracheostomy placed?

How long has the child had the tracheostomy?

Does the child normally need ventilatory assistance at home?

The most probable cause of difficulties is obstruction of the tracheostomy. Obstruction presents with tachypnea, cyanosis, decreased breath sounds, and retractions.

If these children are involved in an accident, make sure that the tracheostomy remains patent and does not become occluded. These children develop true airway emergencies if the tracheostomy becomes occluded and need immediate attention to remove the source of obstruction. Suction and high–flow oxygen are imperative. If suction and oxygen do not improve the status of the child, the child may need the tracheostomy changed. This change should be made en route to the hospital if the provider is qualified to do so. Most parents will have an extra tracheostomy tube at home. If the provider cannot change the tracheostomy, support the child with suction and oxygen and transport rapidly to an appropriate facility.

CENTRAL VENOUS ACCESS DEVICES

Central venous catheterization of the subclavian or other large veins allows the infusion of high–osmolarity solutions into a high–flow venous system, decreasing the likelihood of thrombophlebitis and sclerosis.[6] These access devices are used for chemotherapy and parenteral nutrition, and as a direct line for children with chronic illnesses, such as sickle cell disease, who require frequent IV cannulation.

These catheters come with such names as Broviac, Hickman, and CVL. The placement can be the subclavian or, frequently, the femoral vein in children (Figure D.5).

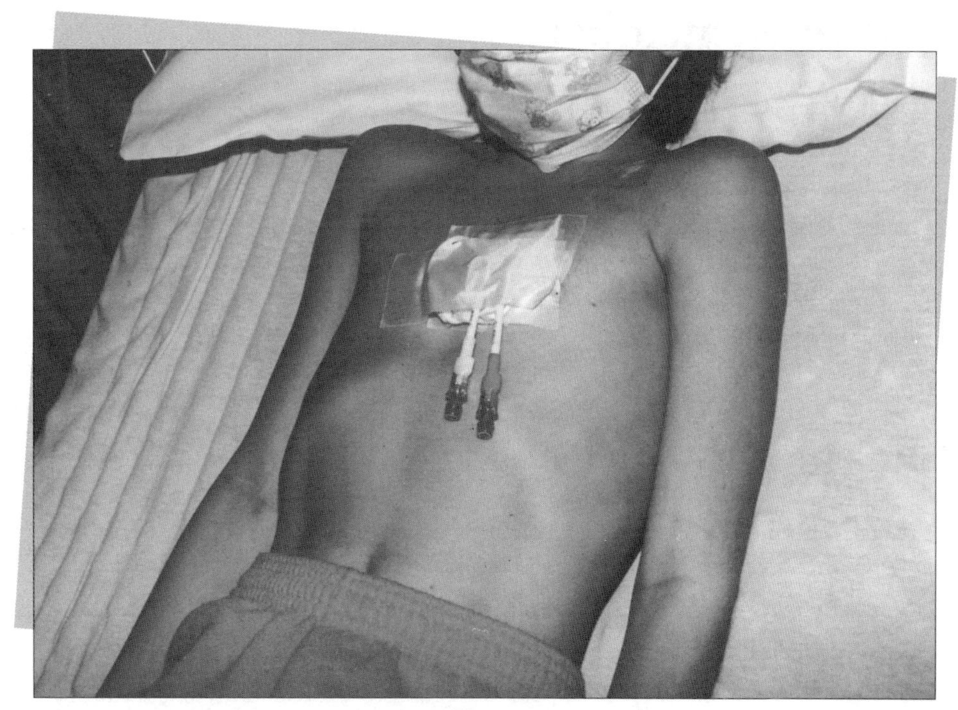

Figure D.5. Picture of a broviac.

Important questions to ask regarding these children are:

Why does the child have the catheter?

When was the catheter placed?

Exsanguination is a major risk factor for children with catheters. If these devices are not taped very well, some children may play with them and even bite them. In the event of a catheter rupture, the clamp given to the family for home use should be used promptly to stop the blood flow and inhibit air and bacterial flow into the catheter. If the family does not have a clamp, hemostats with gauze on the tips can be used to stop the blood flow. Regular hemostats may further tear the catheter. If the catheter falls out, the child will usually not have a significant amount of bleeding. Be sure to apply a dressing. If a child with a catheter is involved in an accident, obtain complete information on the reason for the placement of the device. Most children with catheters have chronic medical problems that may influence trauma care, e.g., a child with hemophilia (a severe bleeding disorder) who is involved in a motor vehicle accident. These children should be transported to the appropriate hospital, with control of any active bleeding.

Points to Remember

1. Any child can be a victim of trauma.
2. Physically, emotionally, and medically challenged children must have their trauma care needs handled by well–trained prehospital care providers.
3. The key to providing care to any injured child with a pre–existing illness is to obtain an accurate history.
4. The parents of an injured child with a pre–existing medical condition can be a very valuable asset to the trauma care team. Use their expertise in your assessment and care.

Bibliography

1. Grismer A. Apnea of prematurity: Current management and nursing implications. *Pediatric Nursing* 1990 Nov/Dec;16(6).
2. Hazinski M. Nursing care of the critically ill child. 1992: Mosby Year Book: 462–3.
3. Dorland's Medical Dictionary 26th edition Saunders 1985 p 622.
4. Fleischer G, Ludwig S. Textbook of Pediatric Emergency Medicine Williams and Wilkins, 1993.
5. Rudolph A. Rudolph's Pediatrics Appleton–Lange 1991, p 1513–4.
6. Hazinski M. Nursing care of the critically ill child. 1992: Mosby Year Book: 763.

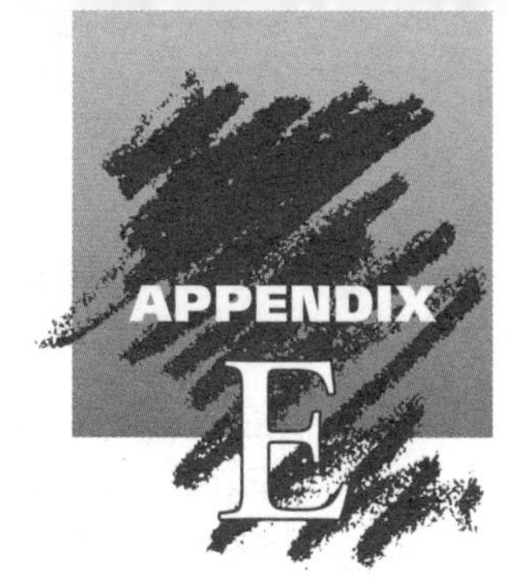

Neonatal Resuscitation

Sharon K. Hammond RN, CEN, EMT–A

Introduction

Trauma extends to all ages. Geriatric trauma is becoming a focus as the country's population ages. The increasing incidence of violent trauma and blunt trauma affects not only the elderly, but the very young as well. Emergency care providers must be ready to deal with a traumatic insult to patients of all ages, even the unborn.

BTLS teaches that the greatest threat to an unborn child is the death of the mother. Care must be directed toward immediate and appropriate management of the mother so that the unborn child will have the best chance for survival. Occasionally, emergency care providers are faced with the delivery of a child in the prehospital setting. This chapter deals with the delivery of a child in the trauma care setting. A delivery of this kind will probably be very unexpected and may be frightening. The chance for survival can be increased if the prehospital care provider understands the basics of neonatal and perinatal resuscitation.

The majority of newborns will need assistance with only temperature control, clearing of their airways, and mild stimulation to maintain adequate ABCs. Occasionally, a neonate will require further assistance, usually after suffering some sort of fetal distress.

Trauma that occurs to a mother during pregnancy may result in fetal distress. Although minor accidents such as falls are common during pregnancy, because of the physical changes that occur to the mother, motor vehicle crashes (blunt trauma) and gunshot wounds (penetrating trauma) not only injure the mother, but also may severely injure the fetus. In blunt trauma, fetal mortality is directly related to maternal mortality. Therefore, aggressive resuscitation of the mother is of great importance.

Blunt trauma to a fetus is more common than penetrating trauma. Minor injuries to the mother may cause fatal injuries to the fetus.[1] One to 5% of fetal deaths are the result of minor blunt trauma. Death from major accidents accounts for 20% to 50% of fetal mortality.[1] Common fetal injuries include skull fractures, chest and abdominal trauma, and premature delivery. Penetrating trauma from gunshot wounds is lethal to the fetus. The mortality rate from gunshot wounds is estimated at 66% and is not directly related to maternal mortality.[2]

ASSESSMENT

When preparing to deliver a neonate after a traumatic injury, prepare to resuscitate an infant in distress. Guidelines from pediatric ALS should be used during the resuscitation. These guidelines should be used when delivering all newborns (Figure E.1).

Be prepared to deliver and resuscitate the newborn. Request additional personnel as necessary. Equipment, including the obstetric kit and the pediatric kit or cart, must be checked regularly to ensure that it is available and ready for use.

The delivery of trauma care to the newborn goes hand–in–hand with initial evaluation and resuscitation efforts.

1. Scene survey
2. Airway, c–spine control, and initial LOC
3. Breathing
4. Circulation
5. Brief exam of abdomen, pelvis, and extremities
6. Critical transport decisions
7. Package and transport interventions
8. Secondary survey

Scene Survey

When called on to take care of a woman in labor, complete your examination while someone prepares the equipment.

It is extremely important to turn the heat on in the vehicle or have a radiant warmer ready to prevent hypothermia, a common complication of the newborn. Carefully extricate the mother if the child has not yet delivered. Consider rapid extrication of the mother if the conditions for delivery will be better in the back of the ambulance.

Three important questions need to be answered before the delivery, if possible: What is the estimated due date? Is there a possibility of multiple births? Is there meconium staining in the amniotic fluid?

The presence of meconium can be detected during an examination of the perineum and indicates that the fetus may be in distress. Meconium is dark–green intestinal material that a neonate may expel if distressed. If meconium is detected, the resuscitation approach will need to change.

Pediatric advanced life support teaches the use of the inverted pyramid as the approach for newborn resuscitation (Figure E.2.). This step–by–step reference should be used with all newborns. Each step should be done within 15 to 30 seconds, and then an assessment or reassessment should be performed. When assessing the newborn, address the ABCs.

NEWBORN RESUSCITATION EQUIPMENT FOR THE EMERGENCY DEPARTMENT (In addition to OB kit)
Gowns, gloves, googles (for universal precautions)
Towels
Heat source (radiant warmer or heating lamps)
Warmed blankets
Suction with manometer
Self-inflating bag (450 mL to 750 mL)
Face Masks (premature, newborn, and infant sizes)
Laryngoscope handles (two) with extra batteries and bulbs
Laryngoscope blades (straight 0 and 1)
Medications and fluids
Epinphrine 1:10 000
Volume expanders (5% albumin, normal saline, lactated Ringer's solution)
Naloxone hydrochloride (1 mg/mL or 0.4mg/mL)
Sodium bicarbonate (0.5 mEq/mL – 4.2% solution)*
Bulb syringe
Meconium aspirator (for attachment to mechanical suction)
Endotracheal tubes (2.5, 3.0, 3.5), two of each
Endotracheal tube stylets
Suction catheters (5F, 8F, and 10F), two of each
Umbilical catheters (3.5F and 5F)
Syringes (1, 3, 10, and 20 mL)
Three-way stopcocks
Feeding tubes (8F and 10F)
Sterile umbilical vessel catheterization tray

* If an 8.4% solution is the only one available, it should be diluted 1:1 with sterile water.

Figure E.1.

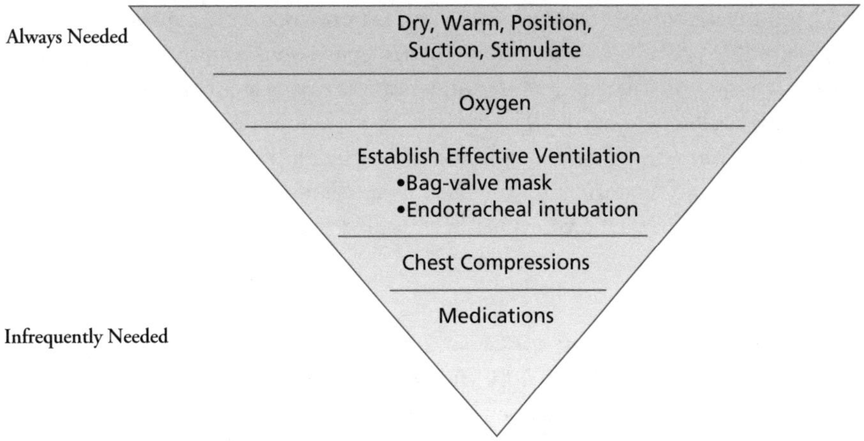

Figure E.2. Inverted pyramid reflecting relative frequencies of neonatal resuscitation efforts for the newborn who does not have meconium-stained amniotic fluid. Note that a majority of newborns respond to simple measures.

Airway and C–spine

If there is a concern about trauma to the newborn, use c–spine precautions. In a standard delivery, this is not a major concern.

The stabilization of the neonate's airway should be of primary concern. *Follow the steps of the pyramid.* First, determine if the newborn is breathing and, if so, whether the breathing is adequate. The normal respiratory rate of a newborn is 40 to 60. Use the color of the child's nailbeds and mucous membranes as an assessment tool but remember that newborns may have peripheral cyanosis, which is normal. When assessing color, look at the face and chest.

Heart rate is the best guide for deciding if the treatments being performed have worked. This can be assessed by palpation at the base of the umbilical cord, femoral or brachial artery, or by auscultation of the apical pulse. In newborns, bradycardia is a sign of an inadequate airway. Correction of the airway problem should result in a normal heart rate of 130 to 180.

The first step in the pyramid is drying, warming, positioning, suction, and tactile stimulation. One of the biggest risks to a newborn is hypothermia. In addition to drying, limit exposure of the body, cover the head, and control the environmental temperature. Position the newborn with a small roll under the shoulders to keep the neck slightly extended. Suctioning may be performed when the head is emerging from the birth canal, but should be repeated again after delivery.

The mouth and then the nose should be suctioned with a bulb syringe. In most newborns, drying, warming, and suctioning will provide enough stimulation to produce a strong respiratory response. Others will require slightly more vigorous stimulation. This is best done by flicking the soles of their feet or rubbing their backs. Reassess for improvement in the heart rate, color, and muscle tone. In newborns, most bradycardia is secondary to an inadequate airway; when the airway has been stabilized, the infant will have an appropriate heart rate.

If the first level of the pyramid is successful, the child will have a strong cry, pink mucous membranes, and good muscle tone. If these attempts fail, the provider should move to the second level of the pyramid, oxygen. Free–flow, "blow–by" oxygen should be provided to a newborn with an adequate respiratory rate and effort and a heart rate of more than 100 who continues to have central pallor or cyanosis. This type of oxygen should be as close to 100% as possible. It can be administered by mask or by placing the oxygen tubing near the child's nose and mouth. The oxygen should be warmed, if possible. Evaluation of respirations, heart rate, and color must continue. Be sure the newborn has been fully dried and is being kept warm.

Breathing

The third level of the pyramid is bag–valve–mask ventilations. Indications for bag–mask ventilations are apnea, heart rate of less than 100, and central cyanosis that does not respond to oxygenation. When assisting ventilations of a newborn, ventilate with 100% oxygen at a rate of 40 to 60. Tidal volumes in newborns will be low. To assess adequate ventilations, observe chest rise and fall and auscultate breath sounds bilaterally at mid–axillary sites. Either an anesthesia or self–inflating type of bag can be used. If the bag being used has a pop–off valve, it should not be allowed to "pop off." Newborns may require higher initial pressures than a pop–off valve will allow.

Because bag–valve–mask ventilations may cause abdominal distention, it may be necessary to place an orogastric tube or light pressure over the abdomen to relieve the distention. After the neonate has been adequately ventilated for 15 to 30 seconds, evaluate the respiratory rate and the heart rate. If the neonate has spontaneous respirations and an adequate heart rate, discontinue bag–valve–mask ventilations and ensure that warming, drying, and stimulation continue.

Circulation

The fourth level of the pyramid calls for chest compressions. Indications for chest compressions are no pulse, heart rate of less than 60, and heart rate of 60 to 80 with no rapid increase following adequate oxygenation and ventilations for 30 seconds. Use standard American Heart Association guidelines for basic life support. Chest compressions are always done in conjunction with bag–valve ventilations. Reassess the heart rate frequently and discontinue compressions when the heart rate is 80 or more.

Pregnancies accompanied by malposition of the placenta may result in increased bleeding at the time of delivery, leading to shock in the newborn. The signs of shock in the newborn are the same as in a child: tachycardia, poor perfusion, poor peripheral pulses, and low blood pressure. To determine a normal blood pressure for a neonate (only if there is time) find out the gestational age of the newborn. The mean arterial pressure of the newborn should be equal to the gestational age. Therefore, a newborn with a gestational age of 35 weeks should have a mean arterial pressure of 35. At this time stop any active sites of bleeding.

Brief neurologic assessment. Neurologic status is difficult to assess in the newborn. In general, the child should be vigorous and have good muscle tone. If the infant is limp, immediately assess the airway. Occasionally, newborns suffer a head injury at the time of delivery; they should be managed in the same manner as a head–injured child.

Critical Transport Decisions

In general, the rules for children apply to neonates. All newborns with an unstable airway, respiratory insufficiency, shock, or an altered mental status require rapid package and transport to the nearest appropriate facility.

Package and Transport Interventions

Airway and c–spine. Endotracheal intubation, the fifth level of the pyramid, should be performed by someone competent with the procedure.

Indications for intubation are when bag–valve–mask ventilations are not effective, when prolonged bag–valve–mask ventilations are necessary, and when tracheal suctioning is necessary, as with thick meconium–stained amniotic fluid. Tube sizes 2.5 to 3.5 are the most commonly used in newborns, depending on their weight. The most commonly used laryngoscope blades are the 0 and 1 straight blades.

Breathing. Endotracheal tube position should be checked initially after placement and reassessed frequently. Placement is best confirmed by auscultation of equal breath sounds and no sounds over the epigastrium. A common complication of intubation in the newborn is right main–stem intubation. After tube placement is confirmed, begin ventilations with 100% oxygen at a rate of 40 to 60 and secure the tube. Assess the heart rate during and after intubation attempts.

Circulation. IV access may be obtained through either the umbilical vein or a peripheral vein en route to the hospital. Use intraosseous access if necessary, but take special care to avoid fracturing the neonate's tiny bones. A smaller (18–gauge) needle may work better than the standard 15– or 16–gauge needle.

Fluid resuscitation may be necessary if there is evidence of hemorrhage and the infant is still pale after oxygenation, the infant has poor or weak pulses despite a good heart rate, or the infant is not responding to resuscitation efforts. Fluid should be given over 5 to 10 minutes. A fluid bolus for newborns is 10 mL/kg of lactated Ringer's or 0.9% normal saline (not the standard 20 mL/kg as in children), 10 mL/kg of a plasma substitute such as albumin/saline solution, or 10 mL/kg of whole blood crossmatched from the mother's blood.

Medications. The final level of the pyramid is medications. The indication for medications in the newborn is a heart rate of less than 80 after adequate ventilation, oxygenation, and compressions have been in place for 30 seconds. The initial resuscitation drug for the infant is epinephrine, 0.01 mg/kg given endotracheally or intravenously. In a prolonged resuscitation, sodium bicarbonate may help reverse metabolic acidosis.

SECONDARY SURVEY

As with all pediatric trauma patients, newborn trauma victims should have a secondary survey completed as time allows. It is important to remember that as a result of blunt trauma to the mother, the newborn may have significant head, chest, or abdominal trauma.

The secondary survey should be done as it would in any pediatric trauma patient. During the initial assessment of the ABCs, initial stabilization is done and the Apgar score is omitted. Once the infant is stabilized, the Apgar scoring may be completed.

SPECIAL SITUATIONS

Meconium Delivery

A special situation in neonatal resuscitation occurs when meconium stains the amniotic fluid. The presence of this thick green particulate matter indicates that the baby has been in distress. Aspiration of this meconium fluid by the infant is dangerous. Meconium–stained fluid is the "exception to the rule" when using the inverted pyramid. It is imperative that such a child not be stimulated following delivery. Suction the trachea under direct visualization with a laryngoscope. Insert the endotracheal tube and attach it to suction as it is withdrawn, removing the meconium. Once the meconium is clear, begin at the top of the pyramid with warming, drying, and stimulation.

Apgar Scores

Apgar scores should not be done on a newborn who requires any type of resuscitation. The wait for 1– and 5–minute scores is too long a delay to determine if the infant needs interventions. Assessments of respiratory rate, heart rate, and color can be done very quickly to establish the need for resuscitation.

Points to Remember

1. Fetal distress can occur due to a number of reasons; one is trauma during pregnancy.
2. Common fetal injuries are skull fractures, chest trauma, and abdominal trauma. Preterm delivery may occur with these types of traumas.
3. The American Heart Association and the American Academy of Pediatrics have set standards of care for the newborn for use in neonatal resuscitation.
4. Be prepared at every delivery to resuscitate the newborn.
5. After the infant is delivered, use of the inverted pyramid will help guide decisions about resuscitation.
6. Meconium–stained fluid is the "exception to the rule." When particulate meconium is noted in the amniotic fluid, use tracheal suctioning and then follow the steps of the inverted pyramid.
7. Apgar scores should not be a priority when a newborn needs resuscitation.

Bibliography

1. Sidky IS, Daikoku NH, Gopal J: Insignificant blunt maternal trauma with lethal fetal outcome: A case report. *Maryland Med J* 1991; 1083–1085.
2. Groff BA, Muntz HG: Gunshot wounds to the gravid uterus: A case report. *J Reproduct Med* 30:4;436–438.

Suggested Reading

1. Chameides et al: *Neonatal Resuscitation. Pediatric Advanced Life Support.* Dallas, American Heart Association, 1990, p 69–75.
2. Campbell JE: Trauma in pregnancy in *Basic Trauma Life Support, Advanced Prehospital Care.* New Jersey, Brady, 1988, p 189–190.
3. Bledsoe BE, Porter RS, Shade BR: *Emergency Management of the Neonate in Paramedic Emergency Care.* New Jersey, Brady, 1991, p 954–971.

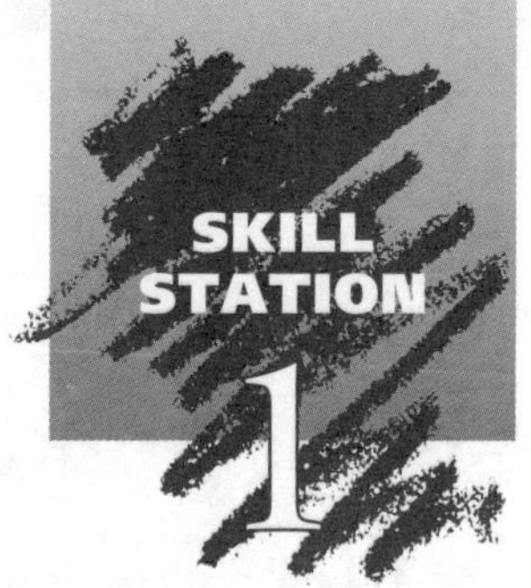

Spinal Immobilization/ Extrication

Objectives

On completion of this station, the participant will be able to:

1. Properly apply an appropriate–size cervical collar
2. Properly log roll a patient onto a spinal immobilization device
3. Properly secure a pediatric patient to a spinal immobilization device
4. Identify which patients should be extricated from a pediatric auto restraint device
5. Perform an extrication of a child from an auto while maintaining c–spine stabilization

SPINAL IMMOBILIZATION

An initial assessment should be performed to identify any life–threatening problems.

Initial Assessment

1. Scene survey
2. Airway, c–spine control, and initial LOC
3. Breathing
4. Circulation
5. Brief exam of abdomen, pelvis, and extremities
6. Critical transport decisions
7. Package and transport interventions
8. Secondary survey

Situations Requiring Spinal Immobilization

1. Mechanism of injury –
   motor vehicle collision, fall, sports
2. Significant injury above the nipple line
3. Head injury
4. Altered mental status (drugs)
5. Distracting injuries
6. Poor historian

If spinal immobilization is needed, the following should be done to ensure maximum immobilization.

Cervical Collar Application

The c–spine immobilization of a child begins with manual immobilization. After the initial assessment has been completed, an appropriate–size cervical collar should be applied (Figure SI.1). The neck should be maintained in a neutral position before and during application.

The patient should be log rolled onto an appropriate spinal immobilization device. Remember to examine the back (Figure SI.2) and allow for the space created by placing the child supine. A folded sheet, towel, or padding may be needed on the board to make up the difference created by the head. The smaller the child, the more padding needed. If log rolling cannot be accomplished, the victim should be pulled onto a spine board using a long axis–type drag. It is extremely difficult to lift a victim without manipulating the spine. Avoid lifting the patient, if possible. The main goal is to place the victim on an immobilization device with minimal spinal movement.

The child should be secured to the immobilization device. The use of straps or other restraining device is necessary to limit the child's movement. Because this is a very frightening procedure, the parent should be involved as much as possible to comfort the child. It is okay for children to be scared. Do not discourage the child or tell him to "be quiet." Comfort the child and explain what you are doing. Immobilize the body, then the head.

The head should be secured to the immobilization device using a cervical immobilization device or towel rolls and tape. Secure the head to prevent lateral movement of the c–spine. The child's c–spine must be stabilized manually until a cervical collar, immobilization device, and head immobilizer are applied.

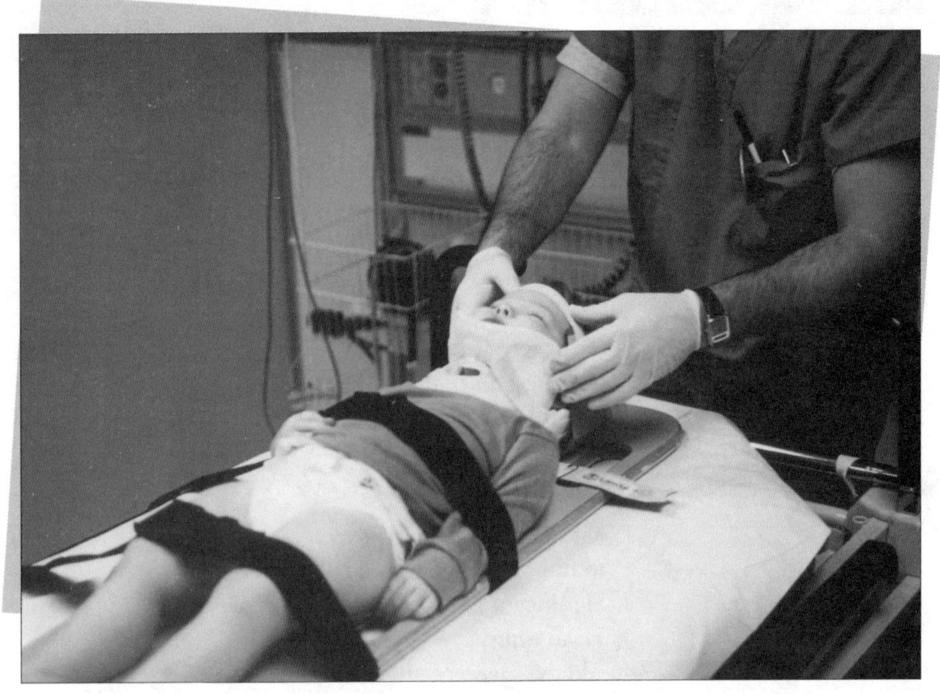

Figure SI.1. Manual c–spine control with a appropriate–size collar.

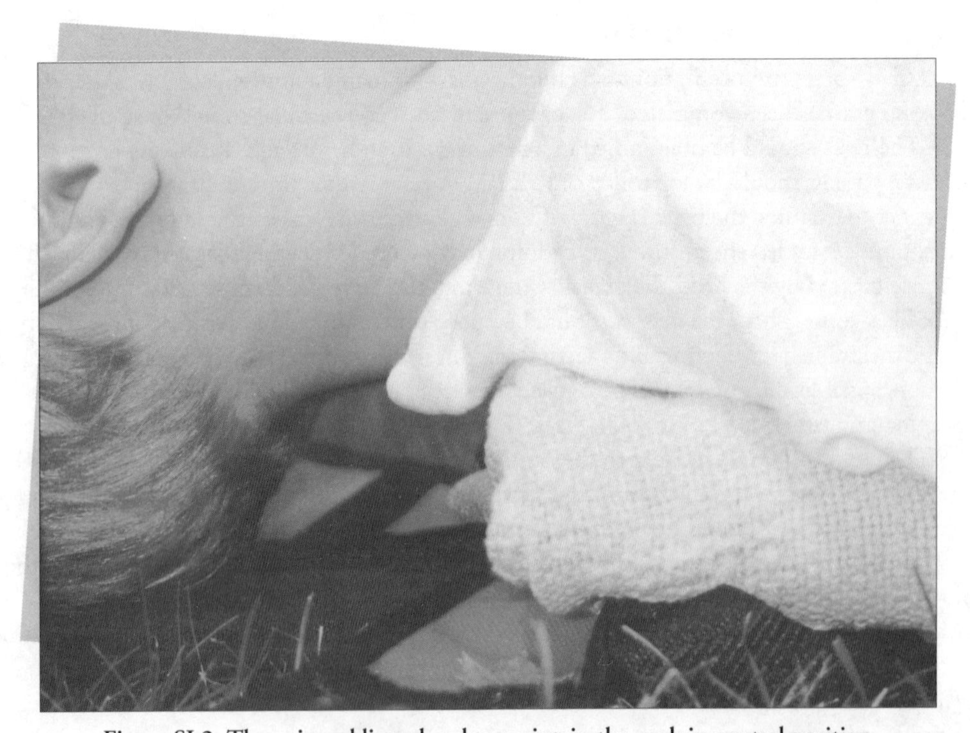

Figure SI.2. Thoracic padding placed to maintain the neck in neutral position.

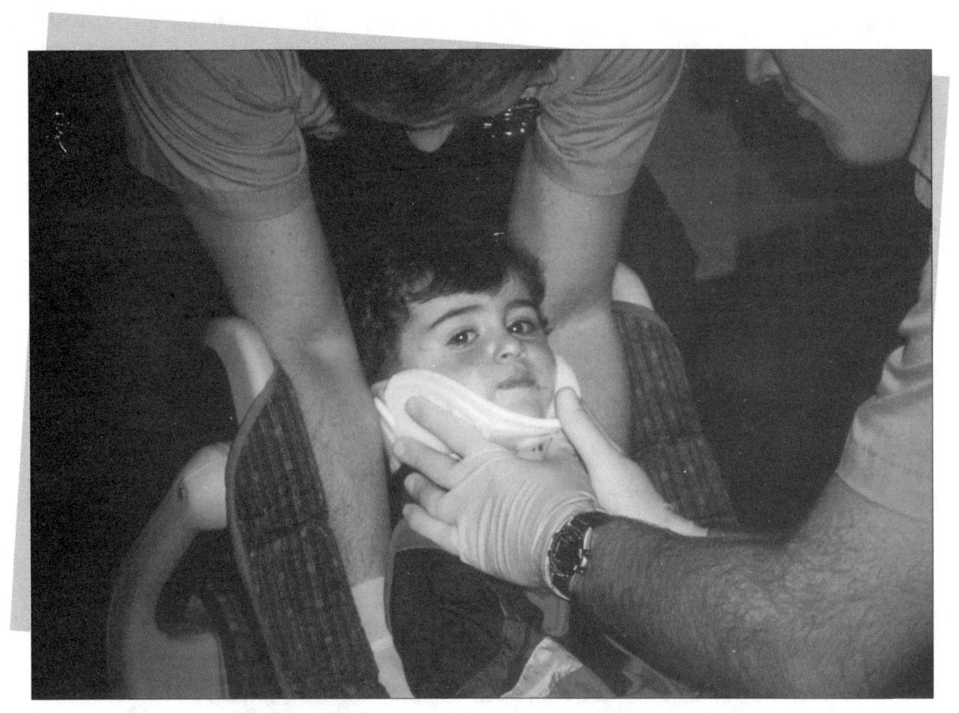

Figure SI.3. Correct placement of a cervical collar.

SELECTING APPROPRIATE EQUIPMENT

Cervical Collar

The cervical collar should fit the child properly. A nonfitting collar may actually worsen a c–spine injury. An appropriately fitting cervical collar will position the child in the "neutral" position, which will decrease any pressure on the spinal cord (Figure SI.3).

Backboards/Pediatric Boards and Straps

After selecting an appropriate–size cervical collar, immobilize the child on a rigid device. The device may be a backboard or other customized pediatric immobilization device. No matter what device is used, it must be used properly. The child must be immobilized in a neutral position. In a small child, a "filler" such as a blanket or foam pad should be placed under the child's shoulder area to align the neck properly. The child should "fit" the board or device. If the child is small and the device is big, the child's "size" must be increased by using blankets so that the child will not move when the board is tilted. The child must be secured to the board with straps or other securing devices to prevent movement. The chest, torso, and extremities must be secured to prevent movement. Usually, a minimum of three straps is needed to accomplish this task (Figure SI.4).

Head Immobilization Device

After the cervical collar and backboard are in place, immobilize the head. This may be accomplished with commercially available devices, cardboard, plastic, or foam; if these are not available, a rolled blanket may be used to secure the head. The head immobilizer must prevent lateral and anterior movement of the c–spine.

Child Passenger Restraint Device

A child found in a car seat should be evaluated. If no abnormalities are noted and the child is in no distress, he may be immobilized in the car seat (the car seat must be removable and intact). A cervical collar should be applied, if possible, and the head should be secured with towel rolls. However, the mechanism of injury may dictate that the child be evaluated at an emergency department. An injured child should be extricated to an immobilization device to prepare for transport. There are no scientific studies showing that immobilization in a car seat is effective; however, if there are no noticeable injuries, this may be an option for emergency medical services personnel.

ARRIVAL AT THE HOSPITAL

After completing a verbal report to the emergency department staff, inform the supervisor in charge that you are leaving your equipment for their use in the emergency department. This will help ensure the return of your equipment. If the equipment is disposable, you may need to inform the emergency department staff of this. If you receive any used equipment, inspect the items closely and clean the equipment as per your infection control policy.

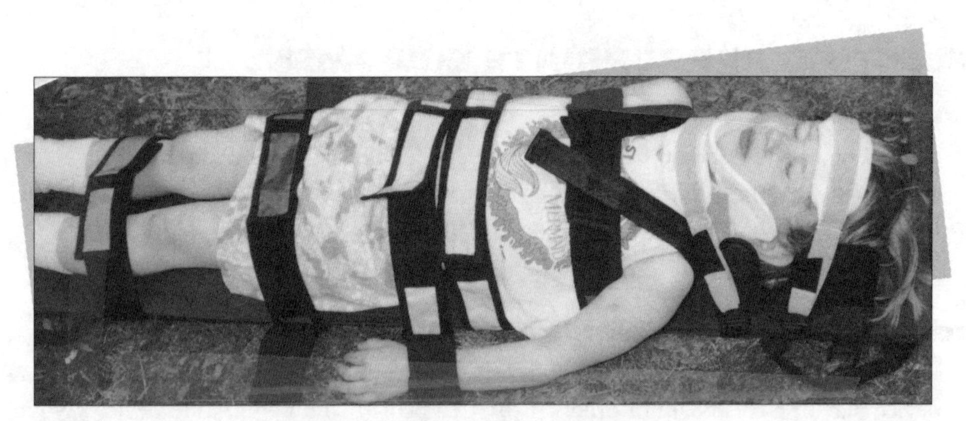

Figure SI.4. Backboard and straps.

EXTRICATION FROM CHILD PASSENGER RESTRAINT DEVICE

Step 1. Evaluate the child to determine if extrication is necessary. If there is any compromise of the ABCs or the child has an altered mental status, the child should be removed to facilitate further examination or interventions.

Step 2. Manually immobilize the c–spine if this has not already been accomplished. It is preferable to extricate the child safety seat if possible, because this preserves spinal protection. However, if the safety seat cannot be moved, Step 3 may be accomplished in the vehicle. Apply a cervical collar if possible.

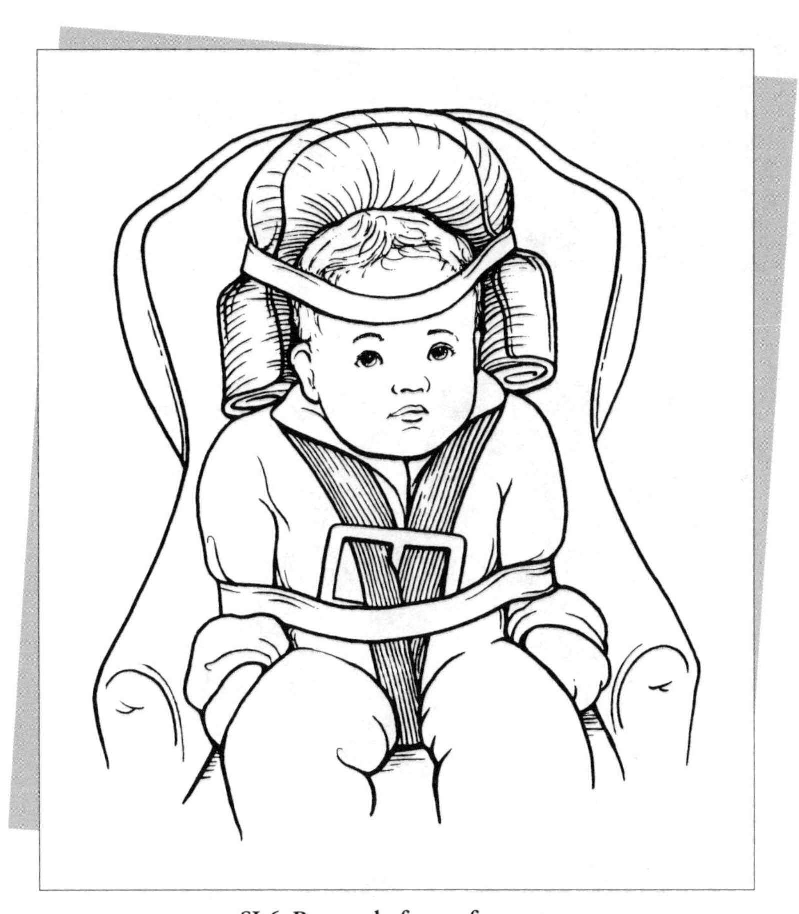

SI.6. Removal of car safety seat.

Step 3. A second rescuer should position himself behind the seat and insert the hands down and under the child and grab the legs. The first rescuer maintains the c–spine. The second rescuer lifts the patient up and out, while a third rescuer places a pediatric immobilization device under the patient. The first rescuer remains in charge of lifting and moving at all times.

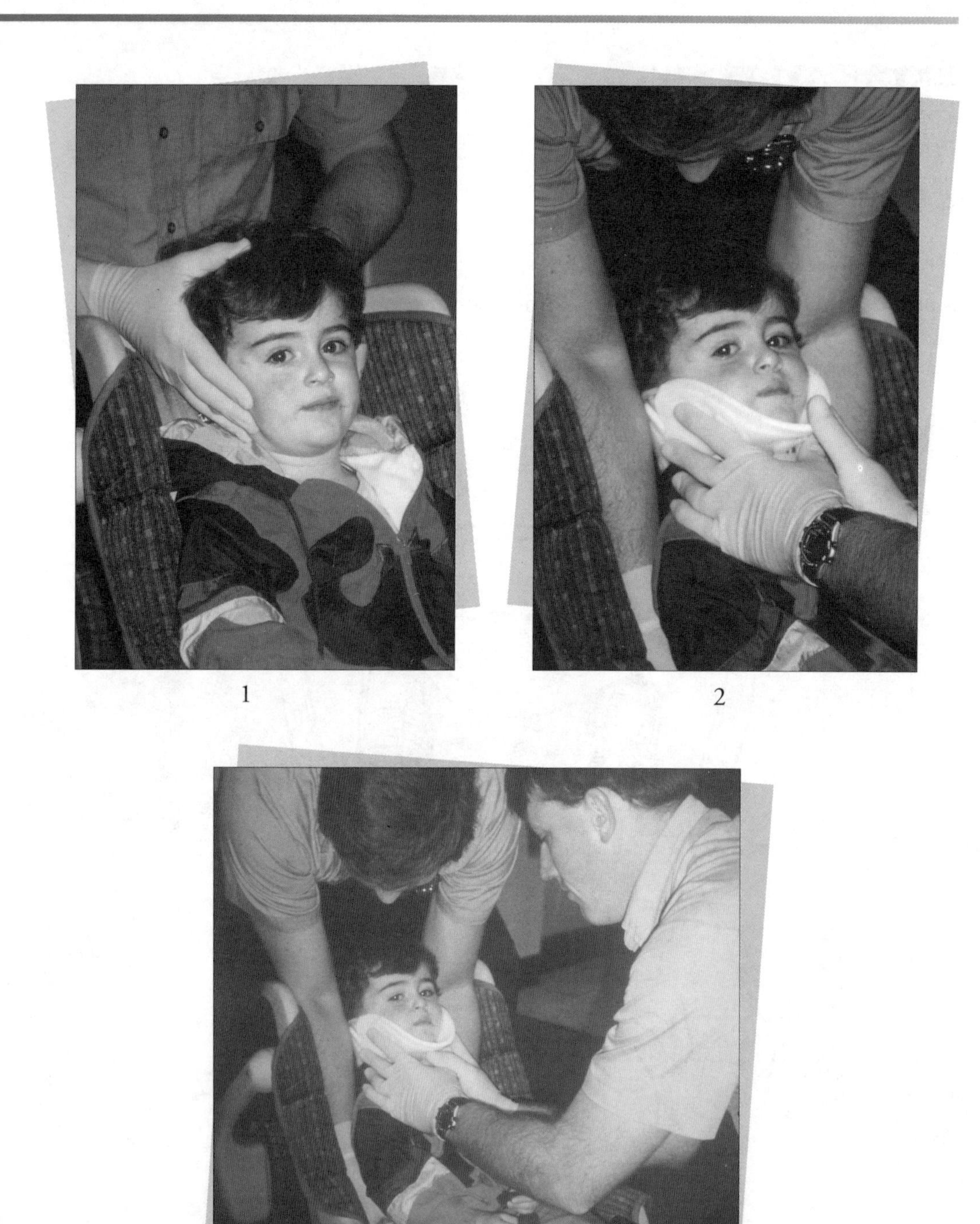

1

2

3

Figure SI.7. Removal of a child from a car seat.

Step 4. The child should be immobilized on the device and moved to the cot in the vehicle as soon as possible.

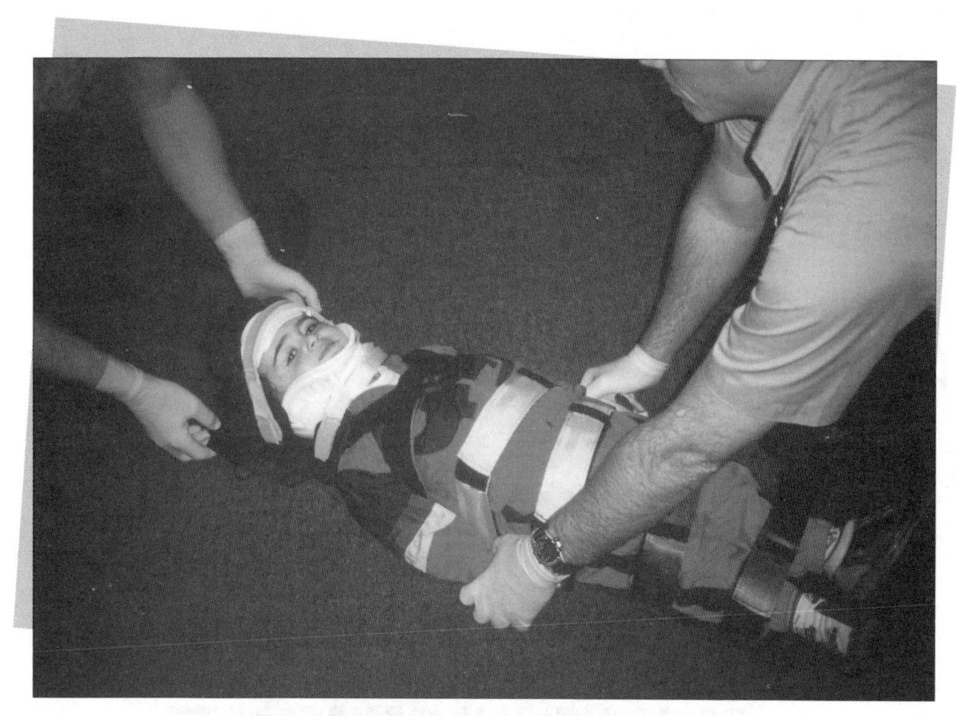

Figure SI.8. Immobilization following removal.

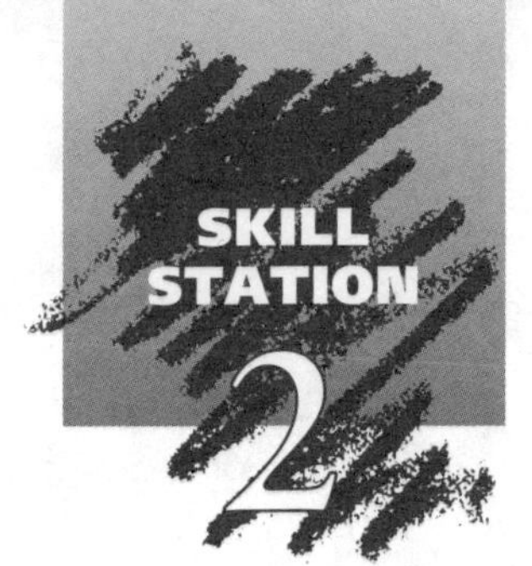

Airway Management and Chest Decompression

BASIC AIRWAY MANAGEMENT

Objectives

On completion of this station, the participant will be able to:

1. Perform an airway assessment
2. Be aware of indications and contraindications for oropharyngeal airways, nasopharyngeal airways, bag–valve–mask ventilations, and intubation
3. Perform bag–valve–mask ventilations successfully

Airway Assessment

After the scene survey has been completed, the patient should be approached and assessed for ABCs, beginning with the airway. The c–spine should be maintained manually in a neutral position, and the patient assessment should begin. If the child can speak in a clear voice or has a normal cry, assume that he has the capability of maintaining a clear airway. This does not ensure that the patient will always be able to maintain that airway, so an assessment must still be done. Examine the oropharynx for signs of foreign objects, bleeding, or loose teeth. Obvious foreign bodies should be removed and the oropharynx suctioned. If the child does not respond verbally, open the airway using the modified jaw thrust. The airway must be examined and suctioned if

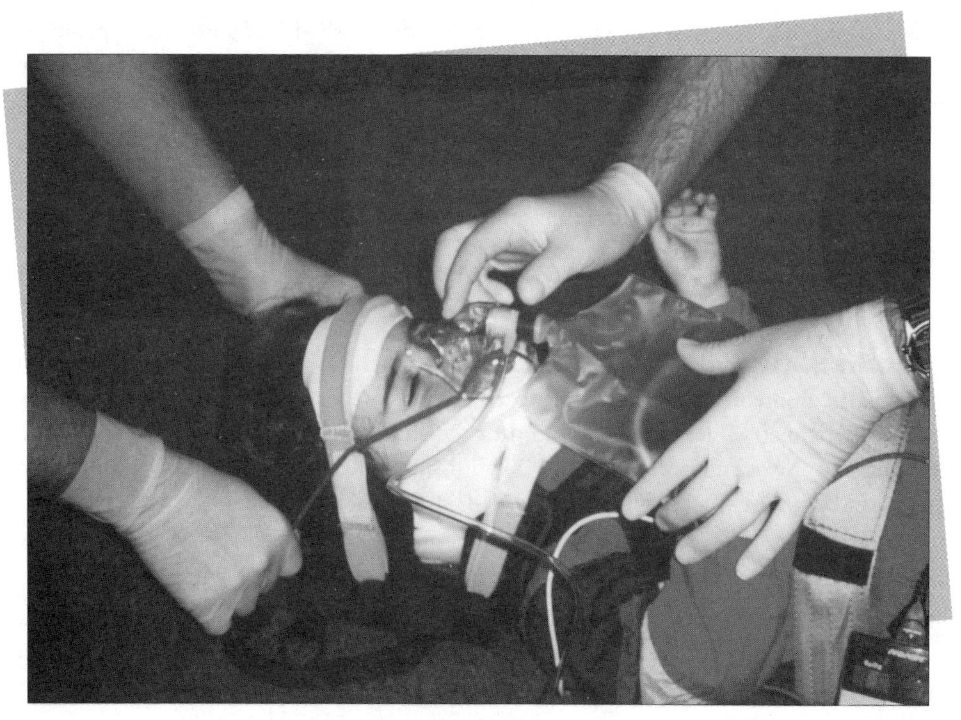

Figure SII.1. Supplemental oxygen.

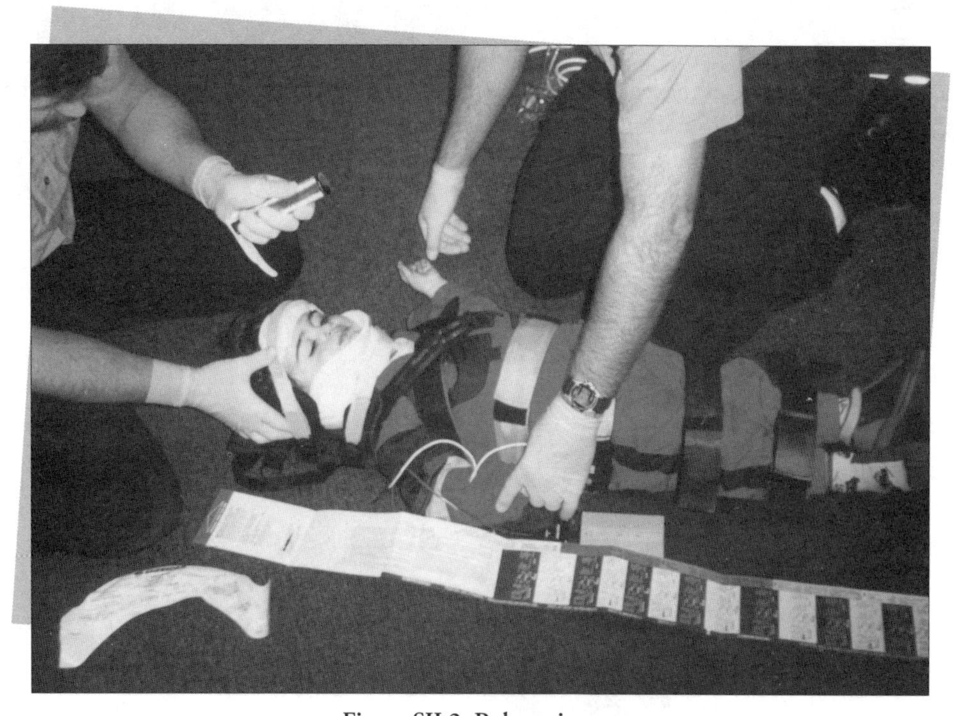

Figure SII.2. Pulse oximetry.

necessary. If the child's level of consciousness remains diminished (Glascow Coma Scale Score less than 8) an artificial airway may need to be established and bag–valve–mask ventilations instituted.

Supplemental Oxygen

Indications. After the determination that a patient can maintain his own airway, administer supplemental oxygen (Figure SII.1).

Contraindications. None.

Method. Oxygen should be delivered to the patient in the highest concentration possible. A pediatric nonrebreather mask at 12 to 15 L/min of oxygen should be placed on the patient. Pulse oximetry may be used to monitor the child's oxygenation (Figure SII.2). The goal is to maintain pulse oximetry readings of 100%. If supplemental oxygen does not maintain oxygenation, bag–valve–mask ventilations with 100% oxygen may be indicated.

Oropharyngeal Airway

Indications. In patients who are unconscious and unable to maintain their own airway, a noninvasive artificial airway such as an oropharyngeal airway may be used. Normally, nasopharyngeal airways are not used due to the small size of the nares and because small children are mouth breathers.

Contraindications. Patients who are awake, because the device may stimulate vomiting.

Method. Correct insertion is critical. Estimate the correct size as shown in Figure SII.3. The phalange should be at the level of the incisors and the tip at the angle of the jaw. The best method for placement is to use a tongue depressor to depress the tongue and insert the oropharyngeal airway (see below and following page).

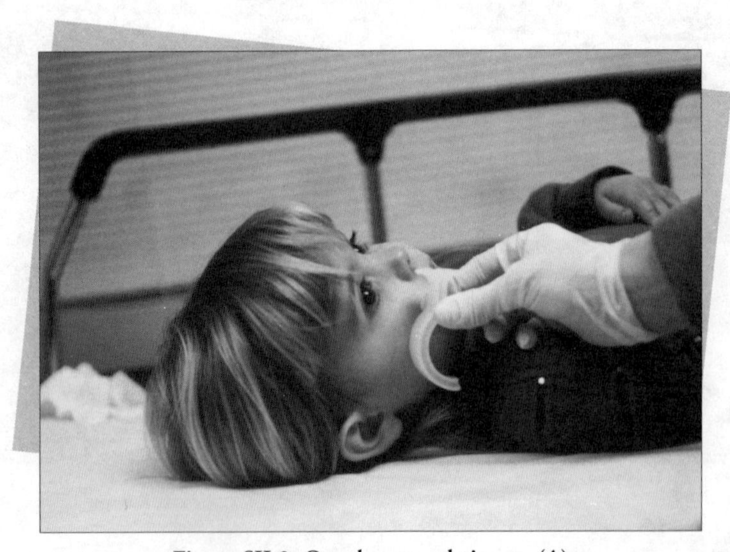

Figure SII.3. Oropharyngeal airway. (A)

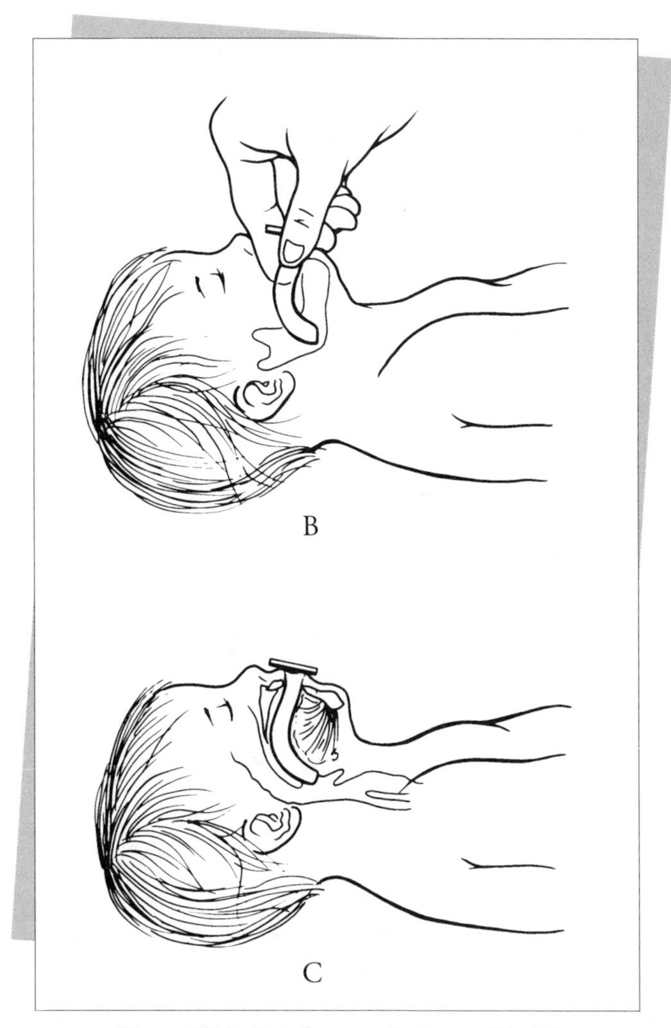

Figure SII.3. Oropharyngeal airway. (B), (C)

Bag–Valve–Mask

Indications. Any child with apnea, inadequate respirations, or severely altered mental status.

Contraindications. Children with upper–airway obstructions should not be assisted until they progress to respiratory failure.

Method. Carefully seal the mask from the bridge of the nose to the cleft of the chin. The mask should cover the nose and mouth, but should not place pressure on the eyes. The mask is held on the face with a one–handed, chin–lift maneuver (Figure SII.4), or in a two–person procedure with one person holding the mask in place and the other ventilating (Figure SII.5). The Sellick maneuver (cricoid pressure) may also be used to minimize the risk of aspiration and the amount of air bagged into the stomach.

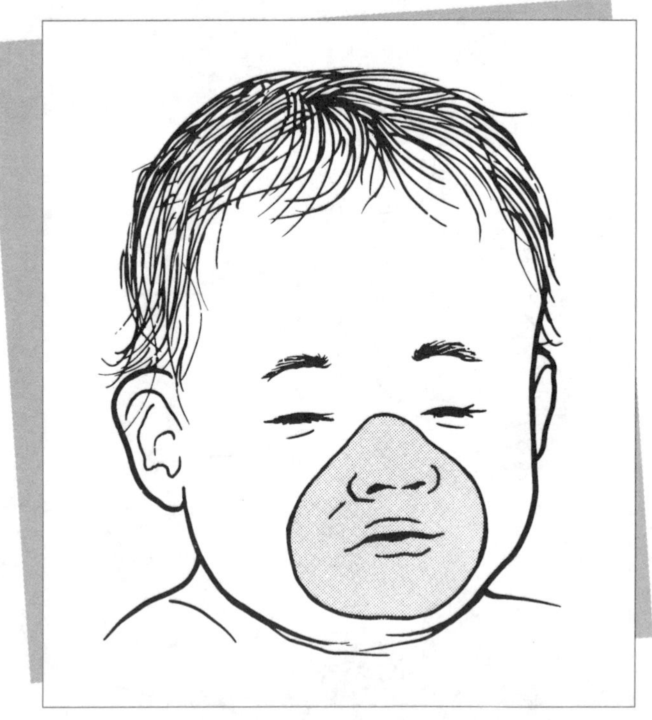

Figure SII.4. Area covered by the face mask.

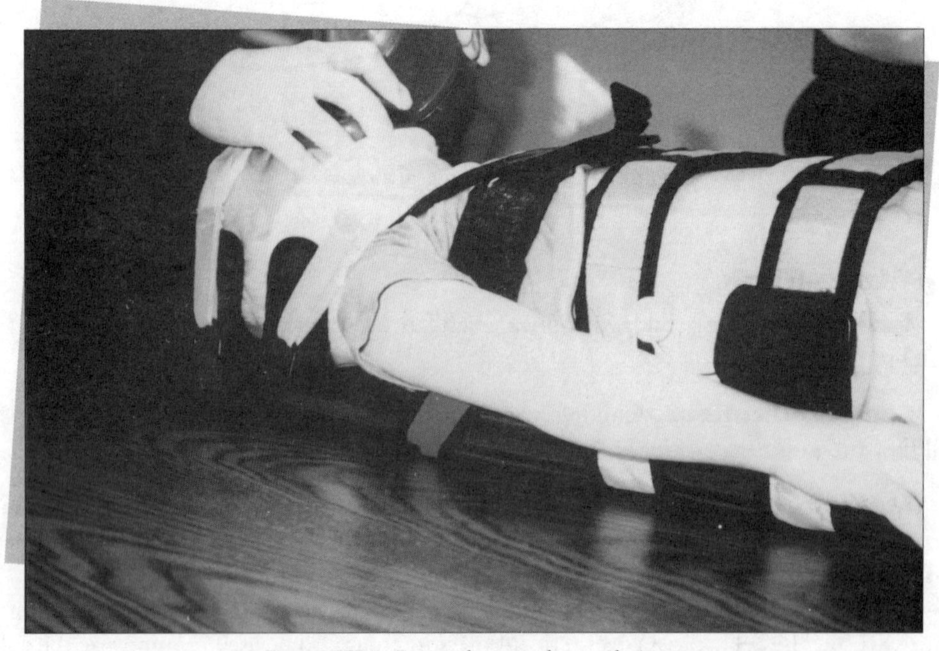

Figure SII.5. Bag–valve–mask ventilations.

ADVANCED AIRWAY MANAGEMENT

Objectives

On completion of this station, the participant will be able to:

1. Perform an endotracheal intubation using in–line c–spine immobilization successfully
2. Be aware of the indications for a needle cricothyroidotomy and a needle decompression

Airway Assessment

When the child is dependent on manual ventilations or can no longer protect his own airway, advanced airway procedures may be needed. The airway should be thoroughly suctioned and bag–valve–mask ventilations begun prior to intubation. If a child is conscious but unable to manage the airway, sedation may be needed before advanced airway manuevers.

Oral Intubation

Indications. Ventilation cannot be achieved with bag–valve–mask ventilations, there is upper–airway protection or neurologic deterioration, or prolonged ventilation is expected.

Contraindications. Combative patient who is maintaining his own airway.

Equipment. Correct–size endotracheal tubes, laryngoscope, appropriate blade, and suction.

Intubation Technique (Figures SII.6 and SII.7).

1. Set up equipment (suction, endotracheal tubes 0.5 smaller and 0.5 larger). Endotracheal tube size may be selected based on a card with values for age, the size of the child's little finger, or the size of the child's nostril.
2. Patient should be ventilated with 100% oxygen before an intubation attempt.
3. A straight blade may be used in the younger child and curved blade in the older child.
4. C–spine immobilization should continue throughout the procedure.
5. The Sellick maneuver may be performed during the intubation.
6. Using the left hand, position the laryngoscope blade at the base of the tongue (straight blade) or in the vallecula above the epiglottis (curved blade).
7. Lift the tip of the blade up and away from you to directly visualize the glottic opening.
8. Insert the tracheal tube from the right corner of the mouth, and insert the tube through the glottic opening.
9. The tube should rest with the two black lines at the vocal cords.

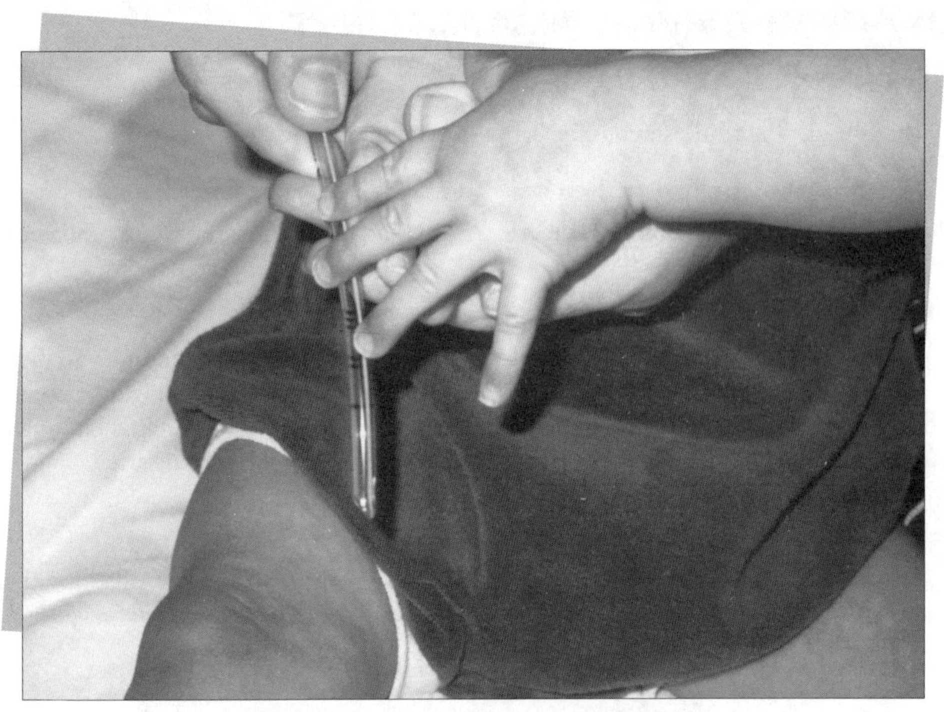

Figure SII.6. Selection of endotracheal tube.

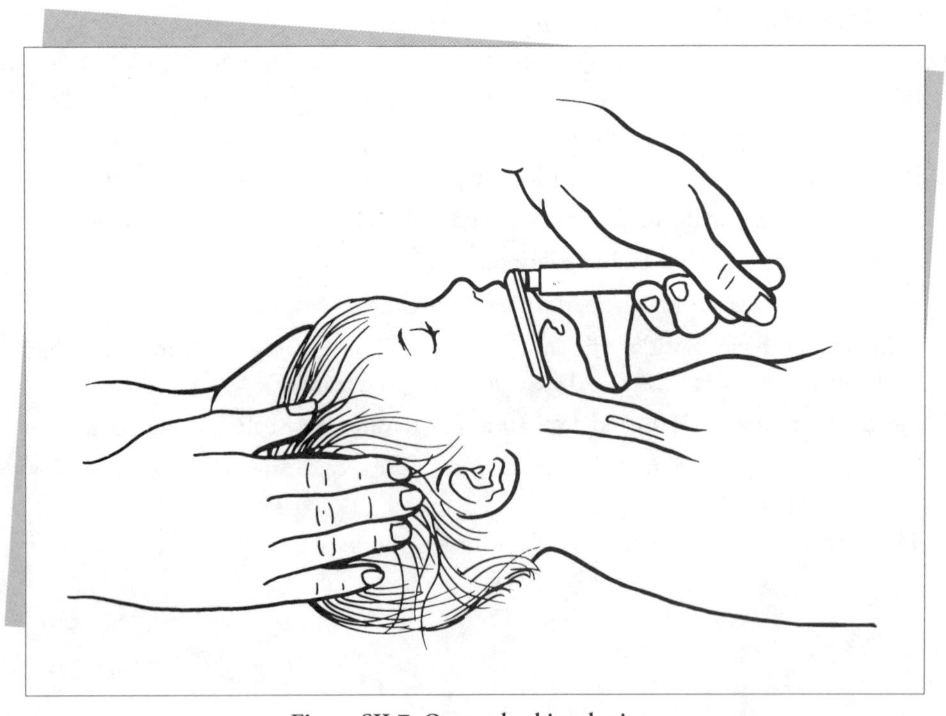

Figure SII.7. Orotracheal intubation.

Confirmation of tube placement.

1. Condensation in the tube during exhalation
2. Symmetrical chest movements
3. Equal breath sounds over both sides
4. Lack of breath sounds over the stomach
5. Improvement in pulse oximetry reading
6. Appropriate response with capnography, or a correct end–tidal CO2 color reading

Blind Nasotracheal Intubation

Blind nasotracheal intubation is usually contraindicated in children. Insertion of an endotracheal tube into the nares has a greater complication rate in children than adults due to the size of the nares and the differences in the anatomy. If orotracheal intubation cannot be accomplished by prehospital providers, bag–valve–mask ventilations are preferred to blind nasotracheal intubation.

Needle Cricothyroidotomy

Indications. Under most circumstances, an adequate airway is provided by repositioning of the head and jaw, an oropharyngeal airway, or endotracheal intubation. Occasionally, a child with an upper–airway foreign body, severe orofacial injuries, or a laryngeal fracture will require this procedure.

Contraindications. This procedure may not be effective in children less than 12 years old because the narrowest part of the airway is the subglottic cricoid ring. *This procedure should be used only in a child who has an obstructed airway in whom all other efforts have failed.*

Equipment. Betadine swab, over–the–needle 14–gauge catheter, and syringe.

Method (Figures SII.8)

1. Palpate cricothyroid membrane anteriorly between thyroid cartilage and cricoid cartilage.
2. If time allows, prep area with Betadine swabs.
3. Use a 14–gauge catheter over–the–needle device with syringe and puncture skin midline and directly over the cricothyroid membrane.
4. Direct needle at 45–degree angle caudally.
5. Insert needle through lower half of cricothyroid membrane. Aspiration of air signifies entry into the tracheal lumen.
6. Withdraw stylet while advancing catheter downward.
7. Attach the catheter needle hub to an IV extension tubing and then to a jet insufflation device (ventilate at l:4 ratio). A second catheter may be needed to allow for exhalation.
8. Auscultate chest for adequate ventilation.

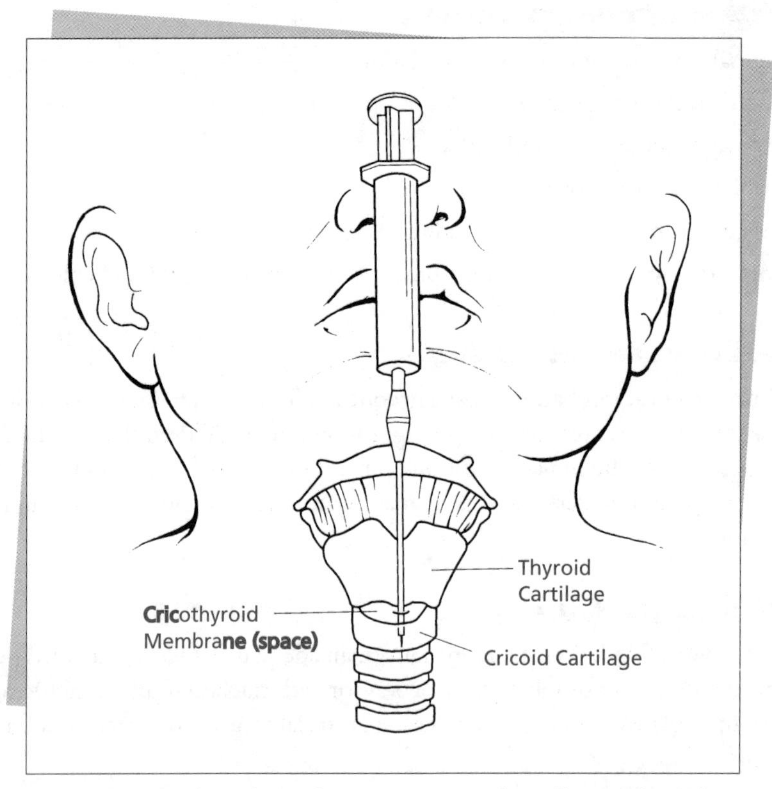

Figure SII.8. Cricothyroid membrane anatomy and needle cricothyroidotomy.

Needle Decompression

Indications. A tension pneumothorax is diagnosed by the combination of severe respiratory distress, decreased breath sounds, and signs of circulatory collapse. Distended neck veins, contralateral tracheal deviation, and ipsilateral hyper–resonance to percussion are not usually present in pediatric cases.

Contraindications. Patients with stable respiratory and circulatory status.

Equipment. Betadine swab, 16– or 18–gauge angiocath, and 30–mL syringe.

Method (Figure SII.9)

1. Administer 100% oxygen to patients with suspected tension pneumothorax.
2. If signs of tension pneumothorax are present, decompression should be accomplished as follows:
   a. Expose entire chest area and clean site vigorously with alcohol or Betadine. Prepare an angiocath (16– to 18–gauge) with 30–mL or 50–mL syringe attached.
   b. Insert angiocath in mid–clavicular line, on affected side into second or third intercostal space. Hit the rib and then slide over it. Thus, the needle should be "walked" upward on the rib until it slides off the upper edge and penetrates into the parietal space.
   c. If air is under tension, it will exit under pressure.

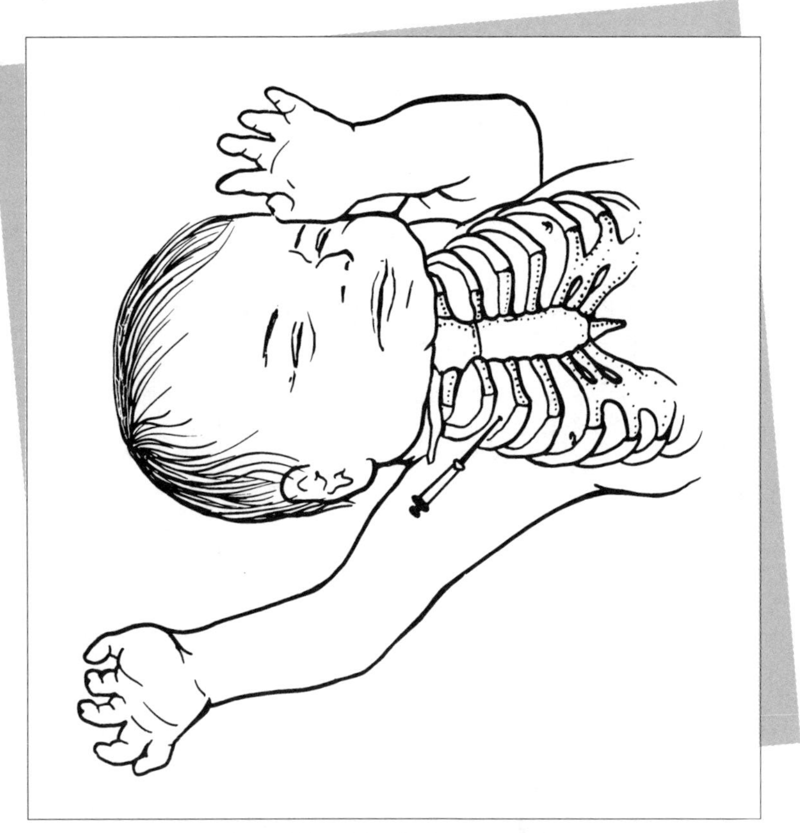

Figure SII.9. Needle decompression.

3. Tape catheter in place. A nonpowdered glove finger may be used to prohibit air re–entry.
4. If no air is obtained, remove needle and cover site with dressing and inform receiving facility of attempt.
5. Continue to reassess adequacy of ventilation.

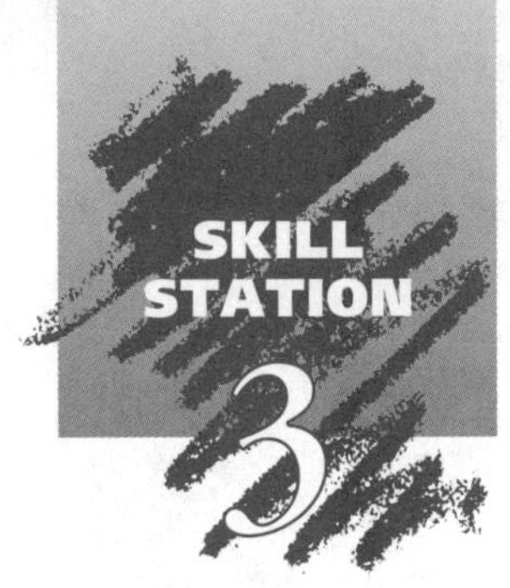

Fluid Resuscitation

Objectives

On completion of this station, the participant will be able to:

1. Identify two sites for peripheral cannulation
2. Demonstrate the technique of intraosseous and peripheral cannulation
3. Describe the indications for intraosseous cannulation
4. Describe how to administer a fluid bolus to a child

INTRAVENOUS ACCESS

Peripheral Cannulation

1. Determine the need for the procedure and obtain permission from medical control or follow–up written protocol.
2. Have all IV equipment ready prior to procedure (over–the–needle catheter, skin cleansing solution, gloves, tape, extremity immobilization board, IV setup).
3. Select a site (Figure SIII.1). Usually the hand or antecubital (preferred) veins are used. Scalp veins are not recommended because the area of the child's head is usually congested with persons facilitating airway management.
4. Immobilize the hand or arm with an arm board and tape in a position of function (Figure SIII.2).

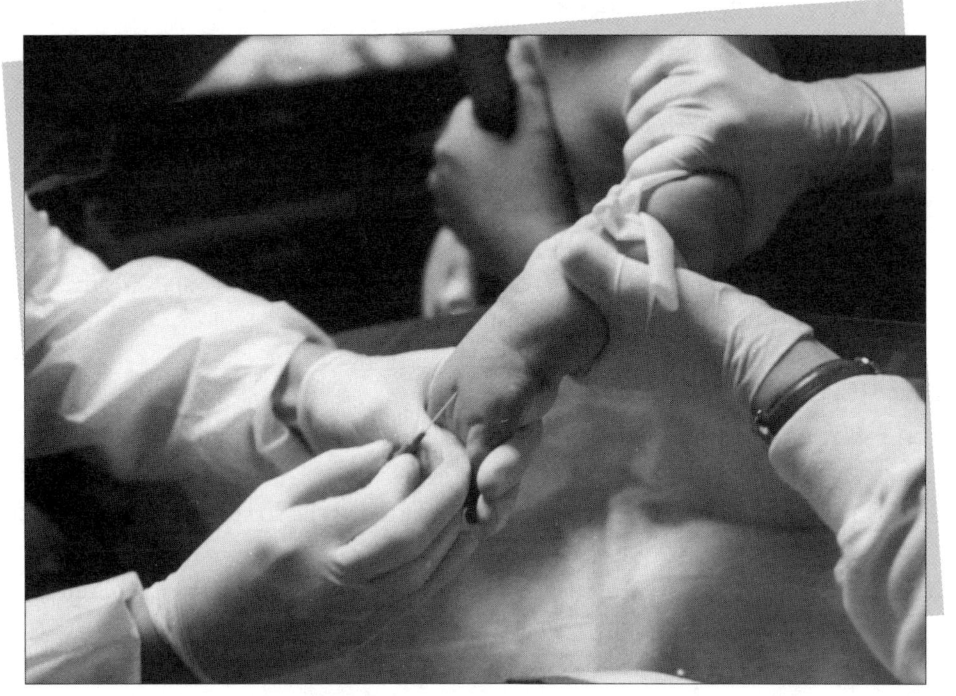

Figure SIII.1. Locating a peripheral vein.

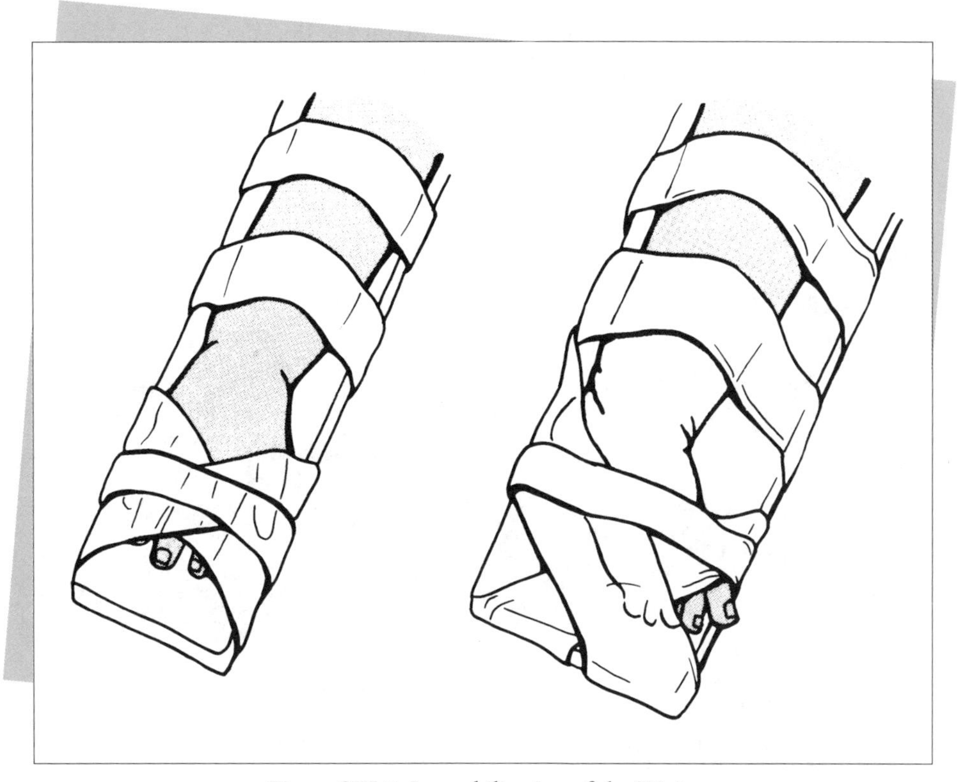

Figure SIII.2. Immobilization of the IV site.

5. Cleanse the site with a cleansing swab.
6. Insert the over–the–needle catheter device (usually a 22–gauge or larger) in the skin and into the vein.
7. Secure with tape, attach standard IV tubing, and infuse fluid and/or medications.

Intraosseous Infusion

The technique of intraosseous infusion of blood, fluid, and medications has been around since the 1930s. The technique re–emerged in the 1980s as a safe, quick, and effective access route, usually for the child who is in extremis.

Indications.

1. A pediatric patient, usually less than 6 years old, who is unconscious and requires fluid, blood, and/or medications.
2. Vascular access cannot be achieved within two attempts or 90 seconds, whichever occurs first.
3. Hypovolemic pediatric patient requiring a transport time of more than 5 minutes and peripheral venous access is unobtainable.

Contraindications.

1. A child with a history of a "brittle–bone" disorder (i.e., osteogenesis imperfecta).
2. An intraosseous needle should not be inserted in an extremity with a recent fracture.
3. If a bone has been stuck once, avoid a second attempt in the same extremity. Fluid, blood, and medications will seep out of the second hole, lessening the infusion of agents to their site of action.

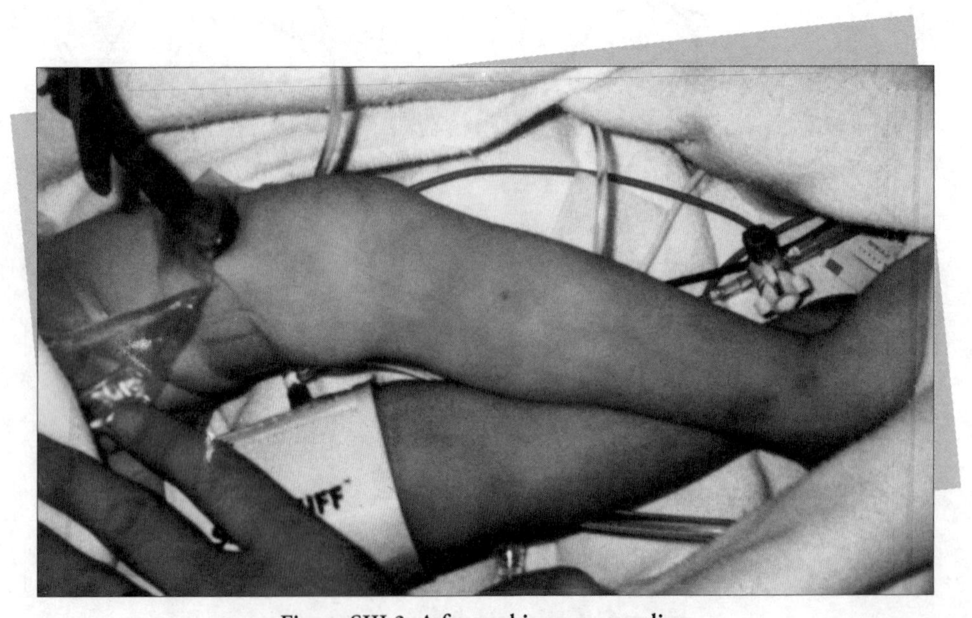

Figure SIII.3. A femoral intraosseous line.

Equipment. Disposable 15– or 16–gauge bone–marrow aspiration needle (18–gauge may be used in small infants), syringe for bone–marrow aspiration, skin cleansing solution, standard IV tubing and syringe with a stopcock, tape, and syringe with flush solution.

Method.

1. Select the site for insertion (Figure SIII.3).
2. The needle is placed perpendicular to the bone with a screwing, to–and–fro motion. Often, a "pop" will be felt as the needle penetrates the bone cortex.
3. At this point, remove the inner stylet and apply a sterile syringe. Aspiration of red marrow fluid (if the child is less than 6 years old) may help confirm placement.
4. Bone marrow should be saved so it can be sent to the laboratory for testing. In the field, the paramedic can obtain a serum blood sugar, an important test in the pediatric patient.
5. Attach a pressure infusion device (e.g., blood pressure cuff) to the bag of fluid to ensure continuous fluid administration.
6. Examine the site frequently for extravasation of fluid and swelling. If these are observed, the needle has been dislodged and requires removal.
7. Secure the needle with tape, and attach standard IV tubing.

FLUID RESUSCITATION

Fluid Bolus Administration

Indications. As indicated in Chapter 6.

Contraindications. Any child who is hemodynamically stable and has pulmonary edema, congestive heart failure, or a severe head injury.

Equipment. Maxi–drip tubing, 3–way stopcock, and 60–mL syringe and extension tubing (Figure SIII.4).

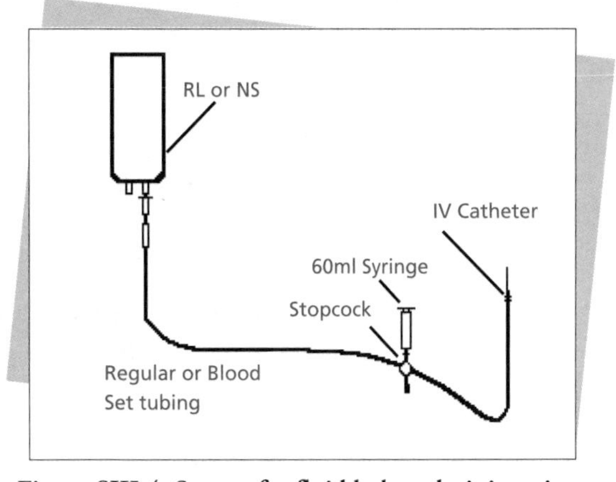

Figure SIII.4. Set–up for fluid bolus administration.

Method.

1. Determine the fluid amount (20 mL/kg) and, with the stopcock turned off to the patient, draw the fluid from the bag into the syringe.
2. Turn off the stopcock to the bag, and, by gentle push, administer the fluid–filled syringe to the child.
3. After the predetermined amount has been given, maintain the IV line at a keep–open rate and reassess the child.
4. Most often, you will notice a dramatic improvement in the child's circulatory status, the pulse will decrease, and the capillary refill will improve. If this does not happen, a second, and possibly third, fluid bolus will be needed.
5. It is imperative that the receiving hospital be aware of the child's response to the fluid bolus as blood products may be required.

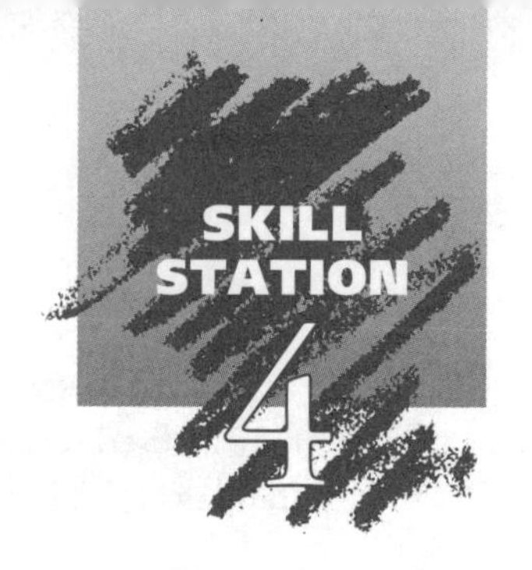

Rapid Patient Assessment

Objectives

On completion of this station, the participant will be able to:

1. Recognize pediatric airway problems
2. Recognize the signs of respiratory distress in a child
3. Recognize the signs of shock in a pediatric patient

ASSESSMENT

Scene Survey

Survey the scene for any hazards and be sure that the team is observing universal precautions.

Airway and C-spine

Take or assign a rescuer c–spine control and establish the level of consciousness. Determine if the airway is open by looking for rise and fall of the chest and listening for exhalation. Use the modified jaw thrust to open the airway. Look for signs of upper airway obstruction, including apnea and stridor. The oropharynx should be suctioned if signs of foreign bodies exist. If the airway is clear and there are inadequate respirations, a bag–valve–mask with 100% oxygen should be used to support respirations.

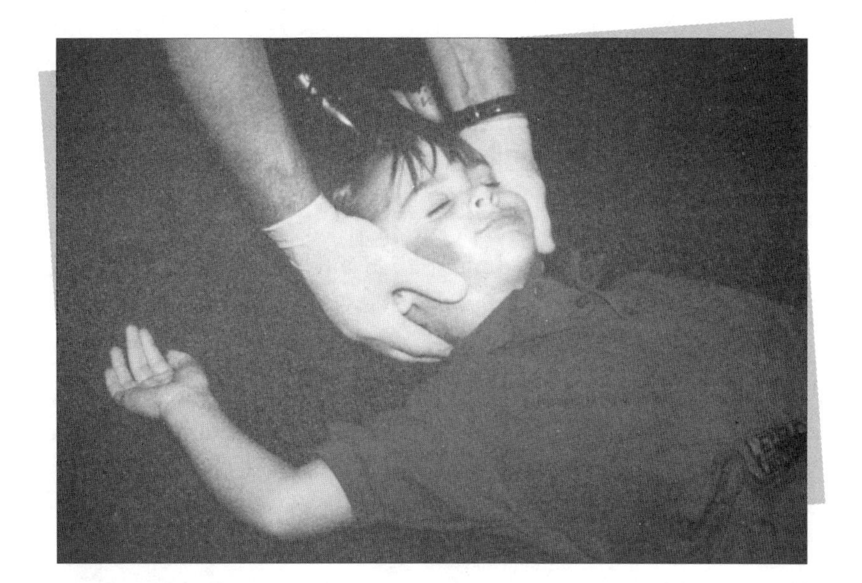

1

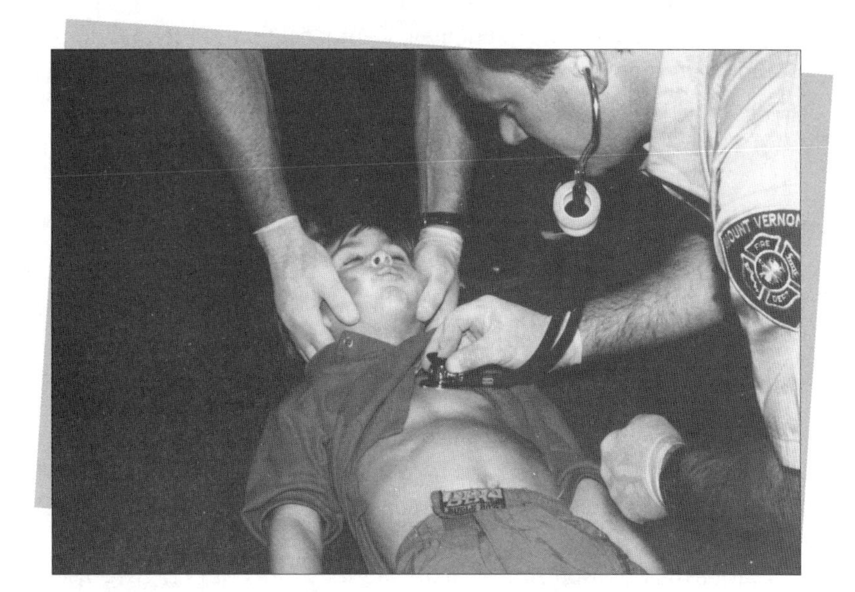

2

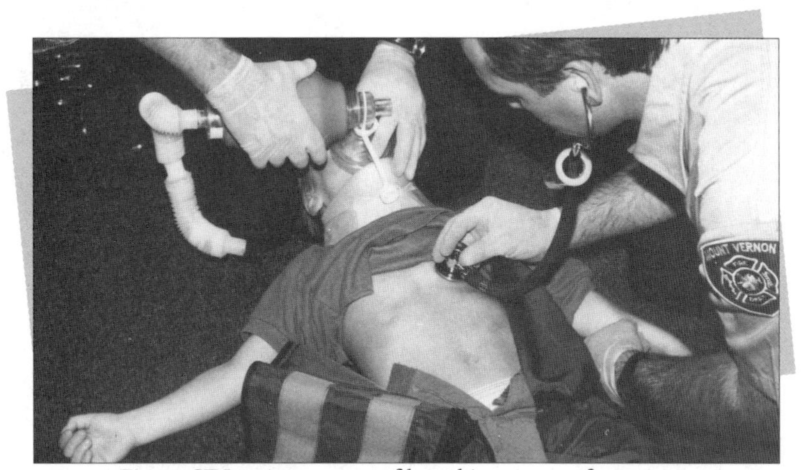

3

Figure SIV.1. Assessment of breathing status of a patient.

Breathing

If not already done, transfer manual c–spine control to a second rescuer and assess for the signs of respiratory distress (Figure SIV.1). Examine the chest and look for symmetrical movement, obvious injury, and signs of respiratory distress, including an increase or decrease in the normal respiratory rate, retractions, or grunting. Auscultate the chest and note anterior and peripheral breath sounds. The trachea and neck veins should also be observed for any abnormality.

Recognize the indications for oxygen administration and bag–valve–mask ventilation and intervene as needed.

Circulation

Assess the circulatory status by taking a peripheral and carotid or femoral pulse. Assess the skin for color and temperature and note capillary refill. Direct a team member to stop any obvious external bleeding. The patient should be exposed to check for any bleeding while body temperature is maintained.

Look for signs of shock (tachycardia, weak peripheral pulses, or poor perfusion).

Quick Survey For Injuries

Rapidly expose and look at the child's abdomen. Gently palpitate all four abdominal quadrants and note any contusions, abrasions, penetrations, or distension. If there is no complaint of pain in the pelvic area, palpitate the pelvis noting any tenderness, instability, or crepitus. The lower extremities should be quickly evaluated for deformity, contusions, abrasions, penetrations, burns, tenderness, lacerations, or swelling.

Brief Neurological Assessment

The level of consciousness should be assessed using the AVPU method: A, alert; V, verbal; P, responsive to pain; and U, unresponsive. It may be difficult to assess the neurologic status of an infant. The parent or guardian may be the best person to help identify changes in behavior (Figure SIV.2).

Critical Transport Decisions

Recognize life–threatening airway, respiratory, or circulatory compromise and any compromise in level of consciousness as a "package and transport" situation.

If there are no immediate compromises noted, perform a secondary examination.

In addition, be aware that transport to a pediatric tertiary care center may be necessary.

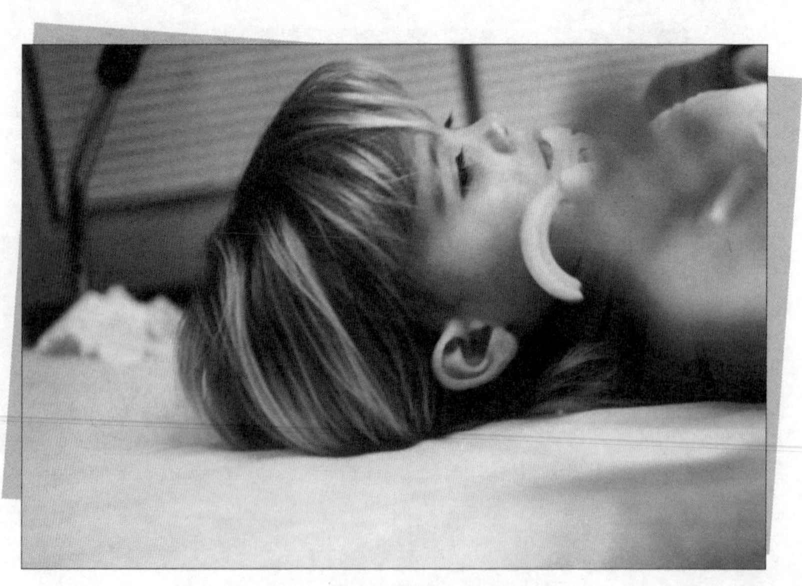

Figure SIV.2

Package and Transport Interventions

Endotracheally intubate the child if bag–valve–mask ventilation is not effective or if the patient's airway cannot be maintained. A needle decompression should be performed if a tension pneumothorax is suspected.

A cervical collar should be applied and 100% oxygen administered. Perform a rapid trauma survey prior to application of the military antishock trousers. The rapid trauma survey should include assessment of the abdomen for any obvious injury, pain, tenderness, rigidity, or guarding. Assess the pelvis for stability and pain. Examine the lower extremities for signs of injury as well as motor, sensory, and vascular status.

Logroll the patient onto a spinal immobilization device. Immobilize the spine keeping the spinal column on a horizonal plane and the midline of the body in alignment. The torso should be secured to the immobilization device first and then the head to allow for minimal movement. Body warmth should be maintained.

Load the patient into the appropriate mode of transportation and depart for the emergency department.

If intubation is necessary, it may be performed during transport. IV or intraosseous access also may be attempted after the airway is secured. Initiate a fluid bolus for signs of shock. A reevaluation of the airway, breathing, and circulatory status should then occur. If time permits, complete a secondary survey.

Secondary Survey

Begin the secondary survey if no life–threatening conditions are found. A secondary survey also may be accomplished in transport after the patient has been packaged and all interventions have been performed. The secondary survey is essentially a head–to–toe examination.

Head assessment. Examine the scalp for lacerations or signs of trauma, including depressions or penetrating objects. Examine the ears for the presence of blood or cerebral spinal fluid. Check the pupils for symmetry. Look for signs of head injury, and examine the nose for the presence of injury, blood, or cerebral spinal fluid.

Neck, chest, and abdomen. Examine the neck for signs of injury, including pain or bleeding. Check the neck veins for distention. A cervical collar may be applied if it is not already in place.

Examine the chest for signs of blunt or penetrating trauma including bleeding or visible injury. Palpate the chest for pain and auscultate. Note the breath sounds, chest movement, symmetry, and effort.

If the patient has already had a rapid trauma survey and the military antishock trousers are inflated, the abdomen, pelvis, and lower extremities may have already been assessed.

If the patient has not had a military antishock trouser survey, assess the abdomen for such signs of blunt or penetrating injury as tenderness, rigidity, and guarding. Palpate the pelvis for stability.

Extremity examination. Examine the lower and upper extremities for such signs of injury as deformity and bleeding, and assess for presence of pulses, sensation, and motor function.

Back examination. Examine the back during the log roll for visible signs of injury. Take a good look as this may be the last time that the entire area will be seen until after surgery.

Neurologic examination. If not already done, conduct a neurologic evaluation and obtain a history. Assess the pupils for equality and reaction to light. Assess the patient (if this has not already been done) for sensation and motor response.

A "SAMPLE" history should also be obtained if possible. This should include S, Symptoms; A, allergies; M, medications; P, past illnesses; L, last meal; E, events of the injury.

Exposure. A thorough examination cannot be accomplished without properly exposing a patient. However, the patient must be kept warm during the process. Passive warming (using warm blankets and hot packs) may be necessary to preserve body temperature.

Packaging for Transport. If the patient exhibits injuries that will need attention at the hospital, package the patient for transport. A cervical collar should be already in place. Log–roll the patient onto a full spinal immobilization device. Secure the patient to the device, and then secure the head using a head immobilization device.

Monitor the patient en route to the hospital. While EKG monitoring may be indicated, monitoring using your hands and eyes is important as well. Reassess the ABCs often.

If the patient requires an advanced airway and no signs of an acute head injury (particularly basilar skull fractures) are present, place a nasogastric tube to relieve gastric distention. If there is any doubt as to presence of acute head injury, place an orogastric tube.

Radio report. A full verbal report should be given to the medical control physician. While some emergency medical service providers operate by written protocols, others will need to establish communications early to obtain permission for procedures. Regardless of the time of contact, the medical control physician will need the following information: unit ID and number, age and sex of patient, chief complaint, method of injury, airway status, respiratory status, circulatory status, vital signs, extent of injuries, and any interventions performed.

Early contact with the receiving facility may be helpful if a trauma team is not available.

SCENARIOS

The student will be given a brief scenario with a moulaged patient and asked to perform a patient assessment. All situations that require a rapid package and transport will be stressed. Each student will take a turn being the team leader. The team leader's performance will be evaluated by the instructor.

Index